119 DAYS TO GO

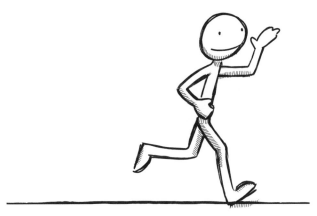

119 DAYS TO GO

HOW TO TRAIN FOR AND SMASH YOUR FIRST MARATHON

CHRIS EVANS

HarperCollins*Publishers*

While the author of this work has made every effort to ensure that the information contained in this book is as accurate and up-to-date as possible at the time of publication, the application of it to particular circumstances depends on many factors. Therefore, it is recommended that readers always consult a qualified specialist for individual advice. This book should not be used as an alternative to seeking specialist advice, which should be sought before any action is taken. The author and publishers cannot be held responsible for any errors and omissions that may be found in the text, or any actions that may be taken by a reader as a result of any reliance on the information contained in the text, which is taken entirely at the reader's own risk.

HarperCollins*Publishers*
1 London Bridge Street
London SE1 9GF

www.harpercollins.co.uk

HarperCollins*Publishers*
1st Floor, Watermarque Building, Ringsend Road
Dublin 4, Ireland

First published by HarperCollins*Publishers* 2021

10 9 8 7 6 5 4 3 2

Text © Chris Evans 2021
Illustrations © Sarah Leuzzi 2021
Design by Louise Leffler

Chris Evans asserts the moral right to be identified
as the author of this work

A catalogue record of this book is available from
the British Library

ISBN 978-0-00-848075-2

Printed and bound in Great Britain by Bell & Bain Ltd, Glasgow

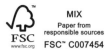

MIX
Paper from
responsible sources
FSC™ C007454

This book is produced from independently certified FSC™ paper
to ensure responsible forest management.

For more information visit: www.harpercollins.co.uk/green

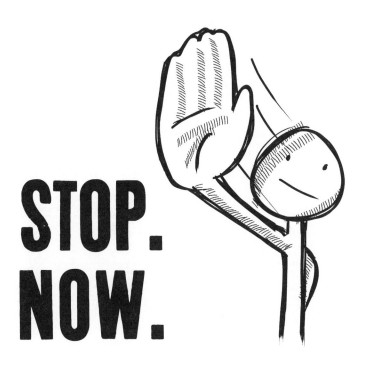

STOP.
NOW.

You have to stop now.
For your own sake.
And for the sake of those you love.
Even for the sake of those you don't love.
You have to stop.
Everything you're doing.
To make your life better.
To make your life yours again.
To give yourself the space and time to be.
Stop.
Now.
Stop everything.

EXCEPT FOR ONE THING.

Don't, whatever you do, stop reading this book.

WAKING UP AND JUST CARRYING ON FROM WHERE
WE LEFT OFF THE NIGHT BEFORE IS NOT WHY
WE ARE HERE.

IF WE DON'T SET OUR OWN FRESH AGENDA
EVERY MORNING, WE WILL END UP BEING PART
OF SOMEONE ELSE'S BY LUNCHTIME.

IF WE DON'T STAND FOR SOMETHING,
WE WILL END UP DYING FOR NOTHING.

WE WERE NOT BORN TO WORRY ABOUT PAYING THE RENT.

OUR BRAIN DOESN'T KNOW THE DIFFERENCE BETWEEN
WHAT'S REAL AND WHAT'S IMAGINED.

THE MIND IS A MONKEY MIND,
OUT OF CONTROL ALMOST ALL OF THE TIME.

THERE IS NOTHING TO FEAR OTHER THAN FEAR ITSELF.

NONE OF US ARE GETTING OUT OF THIS ALIVE.

MANY HAVE TRIED BUT THUS FAR THERE HAS BEEN
A FAILURE RATE OF 100 PER CENT.

THE ONLY WAY TO WIN IS IN THIS MOMENT,
IN THE NOW.

IT'S ALL ABOUT THE NOW.

I AM WRITING THIS BOOK NOW.
YOU ARE READING THIS BOOK NOW.
HOPEFULLY, SOMEONE WILL BE BUYING THIS BOOK NOW.
AND NOW. AND NOW. AND NOW ...

Night following day is Nature's greatest gift to us. Her biggest
hint to date on how we might live our lives. Her way of saying,
'TAKE ONE DAY AT A TIME, YOU IDIOTS, CAN'T YOU SEE? THAT'S WHY
I'VE SEPARATED THEM! F.F.S. WHAT IS THERE NOT TO UNDERSTAND?'

Darkness follows light for a reason, otherwise what would be
the point? Nature never does anything without a reason. Nature
is perfect in her planning. She cannot not plan. Not even if
she wanted to. Nature never feels the need to add. Nature never
overdoes it. Nature never gets bored, or impatient, or frustrated.
Nature is our playbook. Or at least, is supposed to be.

But then again, we are Nature. We are not apart from Nature.
We are part of her plan. We are integral to her ongoing
experiment, we are the ultimate lab rats in the theatre of
evolution. We are, and by some margin apparently, the most
intelligent and advanced species on the planet.

Mmm, it doesn't feel like that sometimes.

Nature is the Almighty. Nature is to be awed. Nature is to be
belittled by and beholden to. Nature is the ultimate higher power
who rewards us the instant we do something right and considers
it her maternal responsibility to chastise us when we stuff up.

So, BEARING ALL THAT IN MIND, what might she be trying to tell us
by rewarding anyone who bothers to walk/shuffle/jog/run around her
planet, purely for the sake of it, with a warm, contagious glow
of profound inner fulfilment? Furthermore, to my knowledge, to date,
Nature has yet to lodge a single complaint against any of her sons
and daughters who has dared to complete a marathon. In fact, to the
contrary, I have it on very good authority she thoroughly approves.

She designed us to move, she wants us to move. She wants us to
realise how much extra juice we have in the tank, both mental
and physical. She wants us to appreciate how amazing we are.
We used to have to run for our lives, to hunt in order to survive.
As far as I can see, the reasons may have changed but our need
to run remains.

WELCOME TO THE CLUB

There are those who can and have completed a marathon; there are those who unfortunately can't; and then there's everyone else. I wouldn't go so far as to say I pity the 'everyone else', that would be way too pejorative, but I do feel like they are genuinely missing out. What to do? The thing is, completing a marathon is a bit like having kids; you can talk parenting until you're blue in the face – whatever that means – but unless you actually are a parent you just won't get it. You can't. It's impossible.

To have walked/shuffled/jogged/run a marathon is transformational. It is Zen. The training for which is a gradual decoding programme that unlocks a vault full of your own innate, bespoke superpowers. The kind of self-knowledge and wisdom that, once downloaded onto your inner hard drive, will be at your disposal for the rest of your life. Proof perfect that, if you can get the necessary shit together to pull off this magnificent feat, the future spoils that await far outweigh the toil it takes to acquire them.

And here's the crazy part: to achieve something the vast majority of our species cannot even begin to wrap their heads around really isn't that difficult.

'PROCESS SAVES US FROM THE POVERTY OF OUR INTENTIONS,' says American sculptor, writer and uber-cool septuagenarian Elizabeth King.

I trained for my first marathon in secret. I didn't even tell my wife. She thought I'd spontaneously fallen in love with walking and the great outdoors. As I seemed so much healthier, happier, positive and relaxed, she elected to leave me alone to get on with whatever it was I was doing.

As usual, she was right. I had and have never been happier. I had and have never been healthier. I had and have never spent as much time outdoors in nature. I had never before had access to such a profound and useful perspective on not only my own life but life in general. Training for my marathon fundamentally changed me as a person and I remain changed to this day.

My simple training regime, my own 119 Days of self-discovery, starting from scratch, (quietly) putting one foot in front of the other, culminated in me running down the Mall in central London on 26 April 2015, 26.2 miles (give or take) after I had set off. I could not believe what I had done, and yet totally believed it at the same time. It felt like magic. Because it is magic. And now, abracadabra! Guess what? It's your turn.

NOW LISTEN UP. I WILL SAY THIS ONLY ONCE.

There is nothing preachy whatsoever in this, YOUR MARATHON JOURNAL, but if I could take a moment to underline one specific point/sentiment/notion/thought - one mantra, if you like - it would be this:

> **IF AT ALL POSSIBLE. COMPLETE EVERY SINGLE TRAINING SESSION WITHIN THESE PAGES. YOU DON'T ABSOLUTELY HAVE TO, BUT TRUST ME, COME RACE DAY, THE FEWER GAPS THERE HAVE BEEN IN YOUR PLAN, THE MORE YOU WILL WANT TO KISS YOUR OWN FACE ON THE START LINE.**

I trained more diligently for my first marathon than any marathon since, and I can honestly say, it remains by far my most enjoyable and least difficult as a result. I have trained 'harder' since, and I have even run quicker (not much but a bit), however the simple fact remains that the innocent, calm, humble and respectful way in which I approached that first-ever 17-week training schedule paid off big time. I felt like I was flying for the first nine miles and that I was employing zero effort.

REMEMBER:

YOUR MARATHON DAY IS NOT THE CHALLENGE.

IT IS THE JOYOUS CELEBRATION OF ALL THE
AMAZING EFFORT, COMMITMENT AND MILES YOU HAVE
QUIETLY RACKED UP OVER A CALM AND BEAUTIFULLY
COMPOSED TRAINING SCHEDULE.

YOU WILL HAVE PAID ATTENTION TO YOUR 119 DAYS.

YOU WILL HAVE COMPLETED THIS JOURNAL
EVERY ONE OF THOSE DAYS.

YOU WILL HAVE CLOSED YOUR EYES EACH NIGHT
WITH THAT INNER BULLET-PROOF KNOWLEDGE THAT
YOU HAVE DONE ALL THAT'S REQUIRED TO BECOME
A MARATHONER.

AND HERE'S THE BEST THING:

YOU ALREADY ARE THAT PERSON.

SO WHAT ELSE CAN I TELL YOU?

Well, not much really, except that it's time to get on the horse.

LET'S DO THiS!!

YEE-HA!!

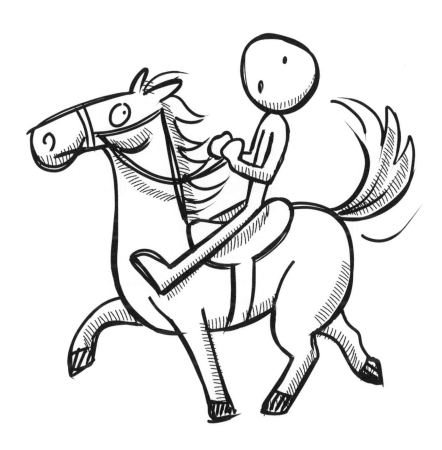

ONLY JOKING.

Not so fast. Like the marathon itself, it's best to start slow and then go even slower. That is, always feel like you have more in the tank. If you feel like you don't have the option to pick up the pace over the next mile, you're already going too fast.

Besides, it's just the best feeling ever to know you have extra reserves of energy, should you need them, while covering distances the likes of which you have previously only dreamt of.

There are precious few afterglows on the planet that come anywhere close to the otherworldly transcendence of the runner's high, and that's exactly where you're heading.

JOURNAL ETIQUETTE

LOVE YOUR JOURNAL. IT IS YOUR FRIEND, YOUR PLAYBOOK, YOUR GUIDE, YOUR INSPIRATION, YOUR TOUCHSTONE.

PLACE IT NEXT TO YOUR BED.

TAP IT FIRST THING IN THE MORNING.

SAY OUT LOUD: 'GOOD MORNING, JOURNAL. HOW ARE YOU TODAY?'

SELECT A REALLY NICE PEN OR PENCIL TO FILL IN YOUR DAILY ENTRIES.

MAKE IT THE LAST THING YOU PUT DOWN BEFORE LIGHTS OFF AT NIGHT.

TAP IT ONCE AGAIN AS YOU DID WHEN YOU WOKE UP.

WHISPER: 'GOODNIGHT, JOURNAL, SEE YOU IN THE MORNING.'

TOP 3 THiNGS TO DO
iN THE FiRST FEW WEEKS

1. Tell people that you are training for a marathon, where it is and when it's happening. This will force you to become ACCOUNTABLE and make your training very real, very quickly.

2. Consider whether you want this to be a SOLO PROJECT or a CO-PRODUCTION. Are you going to train/race alone, with a pal/pals, or a bit of both?

3. Choose AN AMAZING CAUSE to run for. Having a higher purpose (in any aspect of our lives) elevates whatever it is we're doing to a whole new level of CAN DO/CAN'T NOT DO.

ONE MORE THING!

(WELL, ACTUALLY TWO MORE THINGS)

Although I have one hundred per cent written this book – scout's honour, swear down, so help me God and all that other mother jazz – I am not, in any way whatsoever, responsible for the creation and composition of the brilliant training plan within. Oh no, that would be just plain wrong.

All technical aspects of the following training plan have been designed by renowned running guru Dr Martin Yelling. Martin is a former international runner, elite duathlete and triathlete, who also has Hawaii Ironman and Comrades Ultra finishes under his belt. Not too shabby. He's coached thousands of first-time finishers for the London Marathon and is married to two-time Olympic marathon runner and Commonwealth medallist Liz Yelling. He has a PhD in physical-activity promotion and is an experienced endurance coach, writer and presenter, not to mention a dad to three little ones, and the founder of the children's mental health and movement charity Stormbreak.

It was Doc Yelling's beginner's plan that got me to the finish line of my first London Marathon back in 2015. He is my 'go-to' training-plan guy. This time round will be my tenth marathon in his company. He is the man!

When I approached Doc Yelling to create a brand new bespoke plan for a brand new kind of beginner's marathon journal, he didn't hesitate for a second and set to work immediately. What he has come up with as a result is the most thoughtful and comprehensive Yelling wisdom I have witnessed to date.

Doc Yelling, I honour you, I appreciate you, I love you and I owe you BIG TIME.

The only other thing you need to know is the definition of the various different running calibrations mentioned along the way, which are as follows:

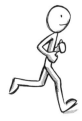

EASY RUNS
50-60 per cent of your maximum effort. These should feel easy and relaxed, breathing should be comfortable and conversation should be easy throughout.

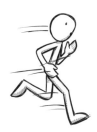

STEADY RUNS
60-70 per cent maximum effort. These will make up the bedrock of your training. Conversation should be more difficult but still possible if not as chatty.

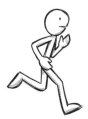

TEMPO RUNS
70-80 per cent maximum effort. These were the ones that confused me at first but that's because I'm stupid. They actually couldn't be simpler. Tempo runs are quite uncomfortable but that's the whole point. They stop you from giving yourself permission to get stuck in a groove of slow or no development.

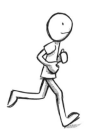

LONG RUNS
These are the holy grail of any marathon plan. They should be revered and respected, embraced and enjoyed. Your long runs are where you will find out who you really are, develop strength and stamina, and figure out that all-important sustainable race-day marathon pace.

Week 1

BLAST OFF!

AT A GLANCE:

Tues: WALK 30 mins

Thurs: WALK/RUN 40 mins

Sat: WALK/RUN 20 mins

Sun: WALK/RUN 50 mins

TOTAL TRAINING TIME:
2 hrs 20 mins

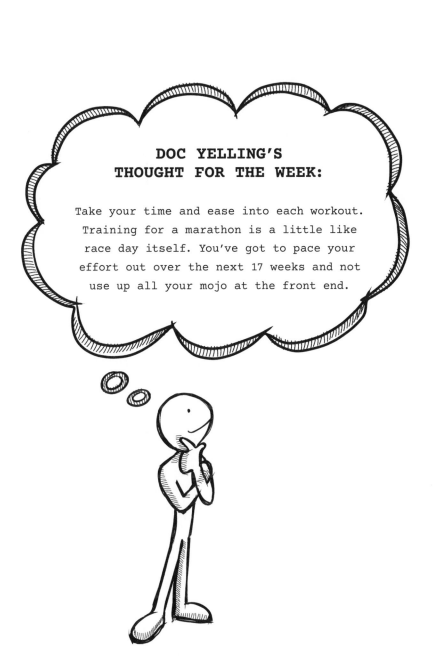

DAY
1

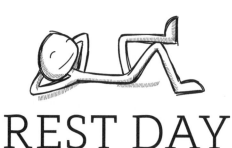

REST DAY

I know! WTF? Day 1, a rest day!!
Go You! You've nailed it! Whoop! Whoop!

INSTEAD OF TRAINING ... TAKE TIME TO CONSIDER YOUR KIT.

When it comes to kit, K.I.S.S. & K.I.L.L.

KEEP IT SUPER SIMPLE & KEEP IT LIGHTER THAN LIGHT.

That is: whatever you like to run in + the minimum of additional
items = making you feel safe, secure, confident and happy.

F.W.I.W. (for what it's worth): I run in really bright running tops
with running tights for all midweek training runs, changing to
running shorts and my race-day race top for all weekend long runs.

The only other items I carry are: an iPod, a credit card, a £20
note and several neatly folded sheets of EMERGENCY LOO ROLL!! All
in a waistband, with the pouch scooched around to the small of my
back. I find this is where it bothers me least. I've tried various
armbands but couldn't get on with them.

I only start to take gels closer to race day. I never take a drink.
I buy drinks en route, as/when/if I need them.

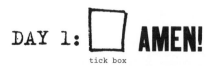

DAY 1: AMEN!

tick box

Week 1: Monday: _ _ /_ _ /_ _

Woke up at: _ _ /_ _ am/pm
In bed now: _ _ /_ _ am/pm

Today I ate: **OK** ☐ WELL ☐ AWESOME ☐
My water intake was: **OK** ☐ GOOD ☐ AWESOME ☐
As a human I was: KIND ☐ THOUGHTFUL ☐ PRESENT ☐

Tomorrow I aim to be 1% better at:

: ....
: ....
: ....

As I prepare to close my eyes
I am grateful for:

: ....
: ....
: ....

pen/pencil down
lights out
3 deep breaths

Only **118** days to go ➡ ➡ ➡ ➡

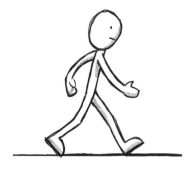

30 mins walk
EASY-PEASY OR WHAT!!

AND WORK THOSE ARMS!

SERIOUSLY, have fun with those arms.

FUN FACT 1: Your arms dictate the speed of your legs, they are nature's accelerator pedal.

FUN FACT 2: You might decide race-walking is the way forward. There's a French bloke who can race-walk a marathon in UNDER 3 HOURS!!

Sacré Bleu! Who needs to run?

Location: ....

Weather: ....

Time start: _ _ /_ _ am/pm

Time finish: _ _ /_ _ am/pm

DAY 2:

tick box

ALL RiGHT!

Woke up at: _ _ /_ _ am/pm
In bed now: _ _ /_ _ am/pm

Today I ate: OK ☐ WELL ☐ AWESOME ☐
My water intake was: OK ☐ GOOD ☐ AWESOME ☐
As a human I was: KIND ☐ THOUGHTFUL ☐ PRESENT ☐

Tomorrow I aim to be 1% better at:

: ....
: ....
: ....

As I prepare to close my eyes
I am grateful for:

: ....
: ....
: ....

pen/pencil down
lights out
3 deep breaths

Only 117 days to go ➡➡➡➡

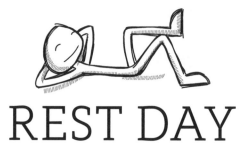

REST DAY

Not again!! I must be joking, right?

Nope, it's another rest day. Whoop! Whoop!

INSTEAD OF TRAINING ...

TAKE TIME TO CONSIDER YOUR RUNNING SHOES.

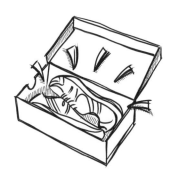

Most decent running shoes are good for approximately 300 to 500 miles. During the next 17 weeks, you'll be covering 200 to 250 miles (WOW! I know, amazing right?) How are yours looking? Would you like to treat yourself to a new pair anyway?

SUPER TIP: If you are going to spend ANY MONEY ON ANYTHING, make it your race-day shoes.

BONUS SUPER TIP: Try to start running in the shoes you intend to run in on race day as soon into your training as possible.

BONUS BONUS SUPER TIP: AVOID CHANGING SHOES ANYWHERE CLOSE TO APPROACHING RACE DAY. Say, no sooner than four weeks to go.

DAY 3: 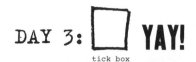 YAY!

tick box

```
┌─────────────────────────────────────────┐
│  Week 1: Wednesday: _ _ /_ _ /_ _        │
└─────────────────────────────────────────┘
```

Woke up at: _ _ /_ _ am/pm
In bed now: _ _ /_ _ am/pm

Today I ate: **OK** ☐ WELL ☐ AWESOME ☐

My water intake was: **OK** ☐ GOOD ☐ AWESOME ☐

As a human I was: KIND ☐ THOUGHTFUL ☐ PRESENT ☐

Tomorrow I aim to be 1% better at:

: ....
: ....
: ....

As I prepare to close my eyes
I am grateful for:

: ....
: ....
: ....

pen/pencil down
lights out
3 deep breaths

Only **116** days to go ➡➡➡➡

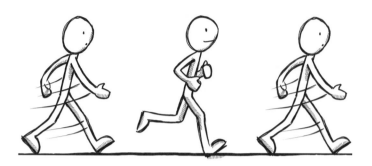

10 mins brisk walk/
20 mins run/
10 mins brisk walk
= **40 mins total**

```
Location:    ........................
Weather:     ........................
Time start:  _ _ /_ _ am/pm
Time finish: _ _ /_ _ am/pm
```

DAY 4: ☐ **BRAVO!**

tick box

Week 1: Thursday: _ _ /_ _ /_ _

Woke up at: _ _ /_ _ am/pm
In bed now: _ _ /_ _ am/pm

Today I ate: OK ☐ WELL ☐ AWESOME ☐
My water intake was: OK ☐ GOOD ☐ AWESOME ☐
As a human I was: KIND ☐ THOUGHTFUL ☐ PRESENT ☐

Tomorrow I aim to be 1% better at:

: ....
: ....
: ....

As I prepare to close my eyes
I am grateful for:

: ....
: ....
: ....

pen/pencil down
lights out
3 deep breaths

Only **115** days to go ➡➡➡➡

DAY
5

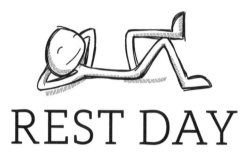

REST DAY

Now you're getting the picture.

For three days a week, you're not going to be running!

FRIDAY RECAP:
What have you decided to do about your race-day running shoes?

F.W.I.W.: I started off running in NIKE shoes for my first few marathons (largely because Paula Radcliffe runs in them and I love her!). I tried VIBRAM FIVEFINGERS for the Amsterdam Marathon, which were fun for a while but a religion I couldn't quite sign up to full time. I had a brief dalliance with ON CLOUD, which felt fantastic to hold, as light as a feather but had this annoying habit of picking up stones in between the ridges on the soles. ASICS always felt too heavy for me. Eventually I fell in love with NEW BALANCE, which are the shoes I still run in now. I'm no expert but I did follow the experts' advice. 'Ignore the advertising budgets and simply choose a reputable shoe that feels most supportive and comfortable for you.'

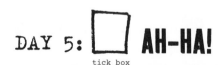

DAY 5: ☐ AH-HA!

tick box

```
Week 1: Friday: _ _ /_ _ /_ _
```

Woke up at: _ _ /_ _ am/pm
In bed now: _ _ /_ _ am/pm

Today I ate: OK ☐ WELL ☐ AWESOME ☐
My water intake was: OK ☐ GOOD ☐ AWESOME ☐
As a human I was: KIND ☐ THOUGHTFUL ☐ PRESENT ☐

Tomorrow I aim to be 1% better at:

: ....
: ....
: ....

As I prepare to close my eyes
I am grateful for:

: ....
: ....
: ....

pen/pencil down
lights out
3 deep breaths

Only **114** days to go ➡ ➡ ➡ ➡

DAY
6

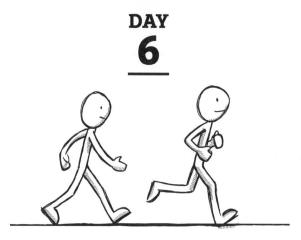

20 mins easy walk/run

OK, THIS IS WHERE THINGS BEGIN TO GET REALLY REALLY COOL AND
EXCITING. YES, ALREADY!!

Saturday training sessions are like training for CHRISTMAS EVE!!
Trust me. The day before your actual marathon, MARATHON EVE, you
will have the kind of feelings you haven't had for years. You will
be TINGLING ALL DAY, raring to go, the wait will be both unbearable
and brilliant. Your INNER CHILD will be irrepressible.

Treat every Saturday between now and then as a dress rehearsal.
STARTING HERE, RIGHT NOW!

Location: ....

Weather: ....

Time start: _ _ /_ _ am/pm

Time finish: _ _ /_ _ am/pm

DAY 6:

☐

tick box

AYE AYE, CAPTAIN!

Week 1: Saturday: _ _ /_ _ /_ _

Woke up at: _ _ /_ _ am/pm
In bed now: _ _ /_ _ am/pm

Today I ate: OK ☐ WELL ☐ AWESOME ☐
My water intake was: OK ☐ GOOD ☐ AWESOME ☐
As a human I was: KIND ☐ THOUGHTFUL ☐ PRESENT ☐

Tomorrow I aim to be 1% better at:

: ....
: ....
: ....

As I prepare to close my eyes
I am grateful for:

: ....
: ....
: ....

pen/pencil down
lights out
3 deep breaths

Only **113** days to go ➡ ➡ ➡ ➡

DAY
7

YOUR FiRST LONG RUN

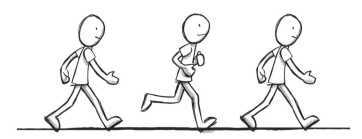

10 mins walk/30 mins easy run/ 10 mins walk = **50 mins total**

Treat your first few long runs as experimental fun runs. PLAY with your routine. PLAY with your routes. PLAY, PLAY, PLAY. These long runs will stay with you forever. They are so special.

EMBRACE the left/right rhythm of putting one foot in front of the other, for a prolonged period of time. This is a tried and tested practice that automatically equalises your breathing, thus helping to engender INNER PEACE, TRANQUILITY, EMPATHY and CLARITY. You get all of these for free when you embark upon one of your long runs.

LONG RUN NUMBER 1

Location: ....
Weather: ....
Time start: _ _ /_ _ am/pm
Time finish: _ _ /_ _ am/pm
Mood before: ....
Mood after: ....

DAY 7:

tick box

KiCKiN' ASS!

Week 1: Sunday: _ _ /_ _ /_ _

NIGHTY NIGHT WEEK 1

Woke up at: _ _ /_ _ am/pm
In bed now: _ _ /_ _ am/pm

This week my diet has been OK ☐ PRETTY GOOD ☐ AWESOME ☐

This week I have slept OK ☐ WELL ☐ AMAZINGLY ☐

This week my training has gone OK ☐ WELL ☐ AWESOMELY ☐

Going into **WEEK 2** I will:

1. Make a decision about my race-day running shoes YES ☐ NO ☐

2. Decide which cause I am going to run for YES ☐ NO ☐

3. Decide whether to run solo or with a pal YES ☐ NO ☐

As I prepare to close my eyes at the
end of WEEK 1, I am grateful for:

1 ....

2 ....

3 ....

Next week in my training I aim to be
1 PER CENT better at:

....

pen/pencil down, lights out, 3 deep breaths

WEEK 1 OFFiCiALLY SMASHED

tick box

Week 2

YOU GOT THiS!

AT A GLANCE:

Tues: WALK/RUN 40 mins

Thurs: WALK/RUN 50 mins

Sat: WALK/RUN 30 mins

Sun: WALK/RUN 65 mins

TOTAL TRAINING TIME:
3 hrs 5 mins

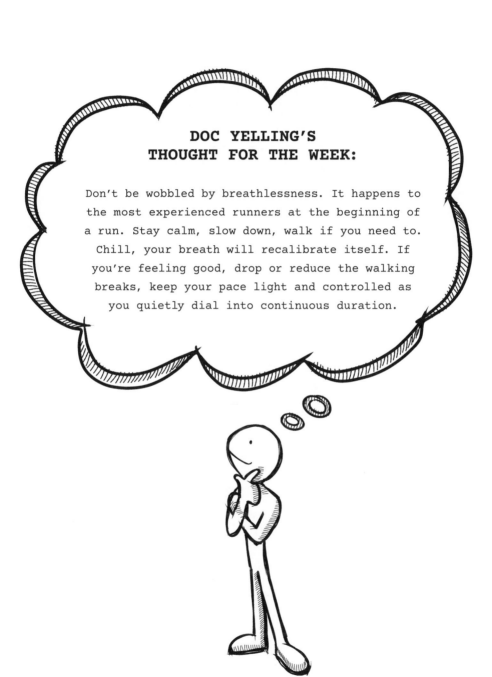

**DOC YELLING'S
THOUGHT FOR THE WEEK:**

Don't be wobbled by breathlessness. It happens to the most experienced runners at the beginning of a run. Stay calm, slow down, walk if you need to. Chill, your breath will recalibrate itself. If you're feeling good, drop or reduce the walking breaks, keep your pace light and controlled as you quietly dial into continuous duration.

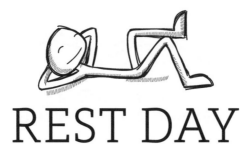

REST DAY

DON'T

THINK

ABOUT RUNNING

OR

ANYTHING

TO

DO

WITH

RUNNING

AT

ALL

(SEE YOU TOMORROW)

DAY 8: ☐ **DONE!**

tick box

Week 2: Monday: _ _ /_ _ /_ _

Woke up at: _ _ /_ _ am/pm
In bed now: _ _ /_ _ am/pm

Today I ate: OK ☐ WELL ☐ AWESOME ☐
My water intake was: OK ☐ GOOD ☐ AWESOME ☐
As a human I was: KIND ☐ THOUGHTFUL ☐ PRESENT ☐

Tomorrow I aim to be 1% better at:

: ....
: ....
: ....

As I prepare to close my eyes
I am grateful for:

: ....
: ....
: ....

pen/pencil down
lights out
3 deep breaths

Only 111 days to go ➡ ➡ ➡

DAY
<u>9</u>

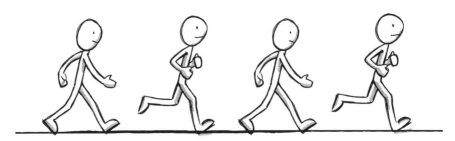

(10 mins walk/10 mins run) x 2
= 40 mins total

FROM NOW ON, ALL THE WAY TO RACE DAY, WEEKDAY TRAINING PAGES WILL
BE SUPER SIMPLE, WITH A SPACE FOR NOTES. DOODLE AWAY!

ALL THE FUN DECISION-MAKING CAN BE LEFT FOR REST DAYS.

THIS IS **YOUR** JOURNAL! ENJOY!

NOTES:

Location: ....

Weather: ....

Time start: _ _ /_ _ am/pm

Time finish: _ _ /_ _ am/pm

DAY 9:

tick box

HALLELUJAH!

```
Week 2: Tuesday: _ _ /_ _ /_ _
```

Woke up at: _ _ /_ _ am/pm
In bed now: _ _ /_ _ am/pm

Today I ate: OK ☐ WELL ☐ AWESOME ☐
My water intake was: OK ☐ GOOD ☐ AWESOME ☐
As a human I was: KIND ☐ THOUGHTFUL ☐ PRESENT ☐

Tomorrow I aim to be 1% better at:

: ....
: ....
: ....

As I prepare to close my eyes
I am grateful for:

: ....
: ....
: ....

pen/pencil down
lights out
3 deep breaths

Only **110** days to go ➡➡➡➡

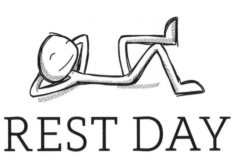

REST DAY

THINK ABOUT SLEEP

SUPER ATHLETES ARE ALSO SUPER SLEEPERS - THIS IS NOT A COINCIDENCE!! Usain Bolt, Roger Federer, Paula Radcliffe, LeBron James, Michael Phelps, Sir Mo Farah .... They all swear by sleep, getting in between 10 AND 12 HOURS A DAY.

SLEEP IS THE SINGLE MOST IMPORTANT THING WE CAN DO TO BOOST/ MAINTAIN OUR WELLBEING AND OUR TRAINING.

Listen to my HOW TO WOW podcast (EPISODE 31) with the sleep guru, MATTHEW WALKER. It's the perfect training listen.

TOP 3 SLEEP HACKS

1: Start trying to go to bed at the same time EVERY NIGHT - EVEN AT WEEKENDS!

2: Create a 'sleep window' of a minimum of nine hours EVERY NIGHT - EVEN AT WEEKENDS!

3: Investigate eye masks and earplugs. You may find them weird at first - I did - but stick with them and you'll reap the benefits.

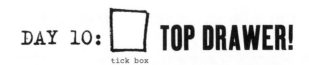

DAY 10: ☐ **TOP DRAWER!**

tick box

Week 2: Wednesday: _ _ /_ _ /_ _

Woke up at: _ _ /_ _ am/pm
In bed now: _ _ /_ _ am/pm

Today I ate: OK ☐ WELL ☐ AWESOME ☐
My water intake was: OK ☐ GOOD ☐ AWESOME ☐
As a human I was: KIND ☐ THOUGHTFUL ☐ PRESENT ☐

Tomorrow I aim to be 1% better at:

: ....
: ....
: ....

As I prepare to close my eyes
I am grateful for:

: ....
: ....
: ....

pen/pencil down
lights out
3 deep breaths

Only **109** days to go ➡ ➡ ➡ ➡

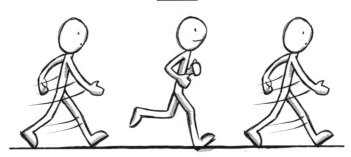

10 mins 'brisk' walk/
30 mins 'easy' run/
10 mins 'brisk' walk
= 50 mins total

NOTES:

```
Location:    .........................
Weather:     .........................
Time start:  _ _ /_ _ am/pm
Time finish: _ _ /_ _ am/pm
```

DAY 11: ☐ **BELLISSIMO!**

tick box

```
Week 2: Thursday: _ _ /_ _ /_ _
```

Woke up at: _ _ /_ _ am/pm
In bed now: _ _ /_ _ am/pm

Today I ate: OK ☐ WELL ☐ AWESOME ☐
My water intake was: OK ☐ GOOD ☐ AWESOME ☐
As a human I was: KIND ☐ THOUGHTFUL ☐ PRESENT ☐

Tomorrow I aim to be 1% better at:

: ....
: ....
: ....

As I prepare to close my eyes
I am grateful for:

: ....
: ....
: ....

pen/pencil down
lights out
3 deep breaths

Only **108** days to go ➡ ➡ ➡ ➡

DAY
12

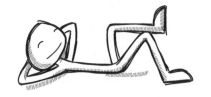

REST DAY

SLEEP (CONTINUED)

5 MORE SUPER SLEEP HACKS

1. Have a warm shower before going to bed, keep your bedroom cool but your feet warm. This killer combo of sleep/heat/prep lowers your body's core temp, which will help you switch off before you drop off.

2. Cut out all caffeine after midday. Caffeine has a half-life of 12 hours!

3. Come off all screens a minimum of half an hour before lights out. Read your journal/listen to a podcast/audio book/calm app/ fantasise! ANYTHING BUT SCREEN TIME.

4. Close your eyes and GIVE THANKS for all that's good in your life, in this moment, right now, and smile as you do so. Don't rush, take your time. LIFE IS SWEET.

5. Practise the SLEEP-BREATHE PATTERN. Breathe in for 5 seconds. Hold for 6 seconds. Exhale for 7 seconds. Pause for 5 seconds. Repeat. This cycle slows down your heart rate and will help your mind and body drift off as one.

SWEET DREAMS.

ZZZZZZZZZzzzzzzzzzz ...　　DAY 12: ☐ **HELLUVA JOB!**

tick box

Week 2: Friday: _ _ /_ _ /_ _

Woke up at: _ _ /_ _ am/pm
In bed now: _ _ /_ _ am/pm

Today I ate: OK ☐ WELL ☐ AWESOME ☐
My water intake was: OK ☐ GOOD ☐ AWESOME ☐
As a human I was: KIND ☐ THOUGHTFUL ☐ PRESENT ☐

Tomorrow I aim to be 1% better at:

: ....
: ....
: ....

As I prepare to close my eyes
I am grateful for:

: ....
: ....
: ....

pen/pencil down
lights out
3 deep breaths

Only **107** days to go ➡ ➡ ➡ ➡

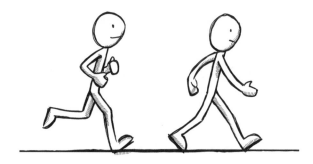

30 mins easy run/walk

ANOTHER BLISSFUL SATURDAY MORNING, ANOTHER DRESS REHEARSAL FOR
YOUR MARATHON EVE.

How are you? How has your week been? What fun route do you fancy
today, ahead of your LONG RUN tomorrow?

I always run on the Thames path on a Saturday. I skip over the
bridge while taking in the day (many deep breaths!). Then I do
something really really naughty. I pick up a coconut flat white
BEFORE I set off! I know. Crazy, eh? Running has made me reframe
and really appreciate the small, simple pleasures in life. They
carry little weight, they don't cost much and I absolutely bloody
love them.

Location: ....

Weather: ....

Time start: _ _ /_ _ am/pm

Time finish: _ _ /_ _ am/pm

Pre-training
treat ....

DAY 13:

[ ]

tick box

ALL GOOD!

Week 2: Saturday: _ _ /_ _ /_ _

Woke up at: _ _ /_ _ am/pm
In bed now: _ _ /_ _ am/pm

Today I ate: **OK** ☐ WELL ☐ AWESOME ☐
My water intake was: **OK** ☐ GOOD ☐ AWESOME ☐
As a human I was: KIND ☐ THOUGHTFUL ☐ PRESENT ☐

Tomorrow I aim to be 1% better at:

: ....
: ....
: ....

As I prepare to close my eyes
I am grateful for:

: ....
: ....
: ....

pen/pencil down
lights out
3 deep breaths

Only **106** days to go ➡ ➡ ➡ ➡

LONG **DAY 14** RUN

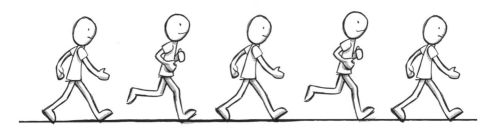

10 mins walk/20 mins easy run/ 10 mins walk/15 mins easy run/ 10 mins walk = **65 mins total**

YOUR SECOND LONG-RUN DAY! Today is an awesome day. BY TONIGHT, you will have officially completed a ONE HOUR+ training run. How @$x*ing COOL is that?

LONG RUN NUMBER 2

Location: ....

Weather: ....

Time start: _ _ /_ _ am/pm

Time finish: _ _ /_ _ am/pm

Mood before: ....

Mood after: ....

WRITE DOWN FIVE WORDS TO DESCRIBE YOUR DAY TODAY:

1. ....
2. ....
3. ....

4. ....
5. ....

DAY 14: 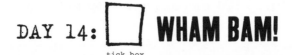 **WHAM BAM!**

tick box

Week 2: Sunday: _ _ /_ _ /_ _

NIGHTY NIGHT WEEK 2

Woke up at: _ _ /_ _ am/pm
In bed now: _ _ /_ _ am/pm

This week my diet has been OK ☐ PRETTY GOOD ☐ AWESOME ☐

This week I have slept OK ☐ WELL ☐ AMAZINGLY ☐

This week my training has gone OK ☐ WELL ☐ AWESOMELY ☐

Going into WEEK 3 I will:

1. Focus on a plan to optimise my quality of sleep YES ☐ NO ☐

2. Listen to the How to Wow podcast featuring sleep guru
Matthew Walker YES ☐ NO ☐

3. Instigate all the sleep hacks mentioned this week YES ☐ NO ☐

As I prepare to close my eyes at the
end of WEEK 2, I am grateful for:

1 ....

2 ....

3 ....

Next week in my training I aim to be
1 PER CENT better at:

....

pen/pencil down, lights out, 3 deep breaths

WEEK 2 OFFiCiALLY SMASHED ☐

tick box

Week 3

LET'S DO THIS!

AT A GLANCE:

Tues: 40 mins WALK/RUN

Thurs: 50 mins WALK/RUN

Sat: 30 mins RUN/WALK

Sun: 80 mins WALK/JOG

TOTAL TRAINING TIME:
3 hrs 20 mins

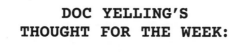

**DOC YELLING'S
THOUGHT FOR THE WEEK:**

This week is about consistency, nailing your
routine and sticking to it. Making your training
regular is the number one super hack that
will make it more likely to happen. Take out
the variables and you take out the needless
(exhausting) decision trees. Get on a roll and
you'll be amazed how much you will look
forward to your runs.

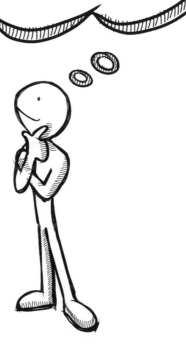

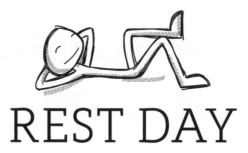

DAY
15

REST DAY

DON'T

THINK

ABOUT RUNNING

OR

ANYTHING

TO

DO

WITH

RUNNING

AT

ALL

(SEE YOU TOMORROW)

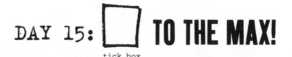

DAY 15: ☐ TO THE MAX!

tick box

Week 3: Monday: _ _ /_ _ /_ _

Woke up at: _ _ /_ _ am/pm
In bed now: _ _ /_ _ am/pm

Today I ate: **OK** ☐ WELL ☐ AWESOME ☐
My water intake was: **OK** ☐ GOOD ☐ AWESOME ☐
As a human I was: KIND ☐ THOUGHTFUL ☐ PRESENT ☐

Tomorrow I aim to be 1% better at:

: ....
: ....
: ....

As I prepare to close my eyes
I am grateful for:

: ....
: ....
: ....

pen/pencil down
lights out
3 deep breaths

Only **104** days to go ➡ ➡ ➡ ➡

DAY
16

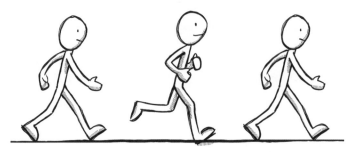

5 mins walk/
30 mins easy run/
5 mins walk
= **40 mins total**

NOTES:

Location: ....

Weather: ....

Time start: _ _ /_ _ am/pm

Time finish: _ _ /_ _ am/pm

DAY 16: ☐ **BOTTOMS UP!**

tick box

Week 3: Tuesday: _ _ /_ _ /_ _

Woke up at: _ _ /_ _ am/pm
In bed now: _ _ /_ _ am/pm

Today I ate: OK ☐ WELL ☐ AWESOME ☐
My water intake was: OK ☐ GOOD ☐ AWESOME ☐
As a human I was: KIND ☐ THOUGHTFUL ☐ PRESENT ☐

Tomorrow I aim to be 1% better at:

: ....
: ....
: ....

As I prepare to close my eyes
I am grateful for:

: ....
: ....
: ....

pen/pencil down
lights out
3 deep breaths

Only **103** days to go ➡ ➡ ➡ ➡

DAY
17

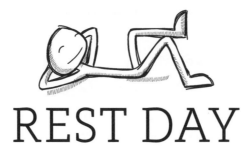

REST DAY

RUNNiNG BUDDiES

If you have decided to buddy up, make sure you take care to choose the kind of company/energy that will enhance your overall experience, as opposed to take away from it. You owe it to yourself to be really honest about this. We are the company we keep. Ditch the sappers, stay with the zappers.

RADIATORS OVER DRAINS!!

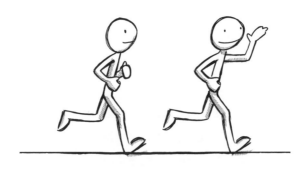

DAY 17: ☐ HOT STUFF!

tick box

```
Week 3: Wednesday: _ _ /_ _ /_ _
```

Woke up at: _ _ /_ _ am/pm
In bed now: _ _ /_ _ am/pm

Today I ate: **OK** ☐ WELL ☐ AWESOME ☐
My water intake was: **OK** ☐ GOOD ☐ AWESOME ☐
As a human I was: KIND ☐ THOUGHTFUL ☐ PRESENT ☐

Tomorrow I aim to be 1% better at:

: ....
: ....
: ....

As I prepare to close my eyes
I am grateful for:

: ....
: ....
: ....

pen/pencil down
lights out
3 deep breaths

Only **102** days to go ➡ ➡ ➡ ➡

DAY
18

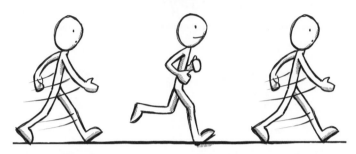

5 mins brisk walk/
40 mins easy run/
5 mins brisk walk
= 50 mins total

NOTES:

Location: ....

Weather: ....

Time start: _ _ /_ _ am/pm

Time finish: _ _ /_ _ am/pm

DAY 18: ☐ **TOP DOG!**

tick box

Woke up at: _ _ /_ _ am/pm
In bed now: _ _ /_ _ am/pm

Today I ate: **OK** ☐ WELL ☐ AWESOME ☐
My water intake was: **OK** ☐ GOOD ☐ AWESOME ☐
As a human I was: KIND ☐ THOUGHTFUL ☐ PRESENT ☐

Tomorrow I aim to be 1% better at:

: ....
: ....
: ....

As I prepare to close my eyes
I am grateful for:

: ....
: ....
: ....

pen/pencil down
lights out
3 deep breaths

Only **101** days to go ➡ ➡ ➡ ➡

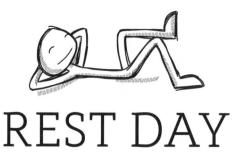

DAY
19

REST DAY

RUNNING BUDDIES (continued)

You may have a pal/pals who are fantastic to work/socialise/play
with and are contemplating training/running your marathon with,
but whatever you do, DON'T COMMIT TO ANYTHING CONCRETE WITHOUT
SECRETLY VETTING THEM. This may sound harsh and extreme, but they
could make or break your whole marathon experience.

TOP 3 CHARACTERS TO AVOID AS POTENTIAL TRAINING PARTNERS

1. Anyone who is too keen to give oxygen to negative thoughts
   while running.
2. Anyone who repeatedly turns up late, disorganised
   and perplexed.
3. Anyone who seems to be much more aggressive and competitive
   than you in their overall approach to running. Or the
   complete opposite: anyone who seems to be too under-ambitious
   and lacklustre for the targets and goals you have in mind.

DECISION THOUGHTS:
Good company rocks but bad company crocks.
It's great to be pushed but don't get crushed.

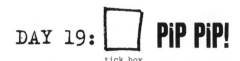

DAY 19:

tick box

PiP PiP!

Week 3: Friday: _ _ /_ _ /_ _

Woke up at: _ _ /_ _ am/pm
In bed now: _ _ /_ _ am/pm

Today I ate: OK ☐ WELL ☐ AWESOME ☐
My water intake was: OK ☐ GOOD ☐ AWESOME ☐
As a human I was: KIND ☐ THOUGHTFUL ☐ PRESENT ☐

Tomorrow I aim to be 1% better at:

: ....
: ....
: ....

As I prepare to close my eyes
I am grateful for:

: ....
: ....
: ....

pen/pencil down
lights out
3 deep breaths

Only **100** days to go ➡ ➡ ➡ ➡

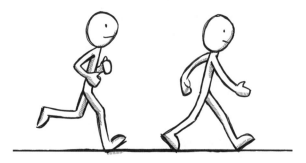

30 mins easy run/walk

CHECK OUT MY SATURDAY/SUNDAY MARATHON TRAINING WAKE-UP ROUTINE:

STAY LYING DOWN. TAKE THREE DEEP BREATHS (OWN THEM, THEY ARE YOURS). GIVE THANKS FOR BEING ABLE TO WALK/JOG/RUN WHEN MILLIONS OF OTHER PEOPLE CAN'T. SPEND A MINUTE MENTALLY VISUALISING YOUR TRAINING ROUTE FOR TODAY AND HOW YOU WANT TO FEEL BEFORE, DURING AND AFTERWARDS. TAKE ONE MORE DEEP BREATH, SWING YOUR FEET OUT OF BED, AND AS THEY TOUCH THE FLOOR SAY OUT LOUD: 'TODAY'S RUN IS GOING TO BE THE BEST/MOST ENJOYABLE EXPERIENCE I CAN POSSIBLY MAKE IT!'

```
Location: .........................
Weather:  .........................
Time start: _ _ /_ _ am/pm
Time finish: _ _ /_ _ am/pm
```

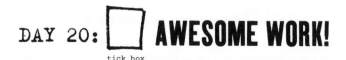

DAY 20: ☐ **AWESOME WORK!**

tick box

Week 3: Saturday: _ _ /_ _ /_ _

Woke up at: _ _ /_ _ am/pm
In bed now: _ _ /_ _ am/pm

Today I ate: **OK** ☐ WELL ☐ AWESOME ☐
My water intake was: **OK** ☐ GOOD ☐ AWESOME ☐
As a human I was: KIND ☐ THOUGHTFUL ☐ PRESENT ☐

Tomorrow I aim to be 1% better at:

: ....
: ....
: ....

As I prepare to close my eyes
I am grateful for:

: ....
: ....
: ....

pen/pencil down
lights out
3 deep breaths

Only **99** days to go ➡➡➡➡

LONG **DAY 21** RUN

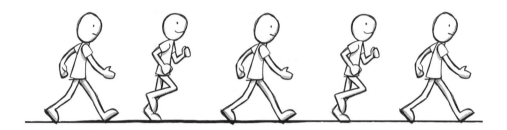

10 mins walk/30 mins jog/
10 mins walk/20 mins jog/
10 mins walk = **80 mins total**

LONG RUN NUMBER 3

Location: ....

Weather: ....

Time start: _ _ /_ _ am/pm

Time finish: _ _ /_ _ am/pm

Mood before: ....

Mood after: ....

WRITE DOWN THREE WORDS TO DESCRIBE YOUR DAY TODAY:

1. ....

2. ....

3. ....

DAY 21: 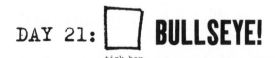 **BULLSEYE!**

tick box

Week 3: Sunday: _ _ /_ _ /_ _

NIGHTY NIGHT WEEK 3

Woke up at: _ _ /_ _ am/pm
In bed now: _ _ /_ _ am/pm

This week my diet has been OK ☐ PRETTY GOOD ☐ AWESOME ☐

This week I have slept OK ☐ WELL ☐ AMAZINGLY ☐

This week my training has gone OK ☐ WELL ☐ AWESOMELY ☐

Going into WEEK 4 I will:

1. Decide whether to train/race with a pal/pals or go solo YES ☐ NO ☐

2. Begin to create a weekend pre-long-run Saturday/long-run Sunday routine YES ☐ NO ☐

3. Check in on my sleep regime YES ☐ NO ☐

As I prepare to close my eyes at the end of WEEK 3, I am grateful for:

1 ....

2 ....

3 ....

Next week in my training I aim to be 1 PER CENT better at:

....

pen/pencil down, lights out, 3 deep breaths

WEEK 3 OFFICIALLY SMASHED ☐

tick box

Week 4

BRRR! WELCOME TO COLD SHOWER WEEK

AT A GLANCE:

Tues: 40 mins WALK/RUN/WALK

Thurs: 55 mins WALK/RUN/WALK

Sat: 40 mins EASY RUN/WALK

Sun: 90 mins WALK/JOG/WALK/JOG/WALK

TOTAL TRAINING TIME: 3 hrs 45 mins

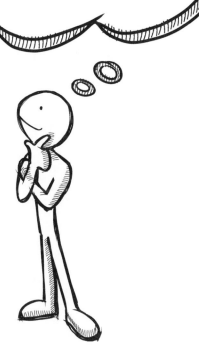

**DOC YELLING'S
THOUGHT FOR THE WEEK:**

Your runs should start to feel easier around now
but beware the ironic subconscious dip in motivation
that can come with that. 'This is easier than I
thought!' NO NO NO. Take a mental cold shower (or an
extended actual cold shower!!!) and reboot whenever you
hear so much as even a whisper of such thoughts.
It's all good. It's all very, very good.
But you must stay on your game.

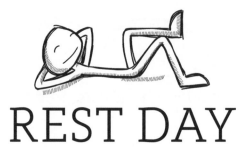

REST DAY

DON'T

THINK

ABOUT RUNNING

OR

ANYTHING

TO

DO

WITH

RUNNING

AT

ALL

(SEE YOU TOMORROW)

DAY 22: ☐ **HATS OFF!**

tick box

Week 4: Monday: _ _ /_ _ /_ _

Woke up at: _ _ /_ _ am/pm
In bed now: _ _ /_ _ am/pm

Today I ate: OK ☐ WELL ☐ AWESOME ☐
My water intake was: OK ☐ GOOD ☐ AWESOME ☐
As a human I was: KIND ☐ THOUGHTFUL ☐ PRESENT ☐

Tomorrow I aim to be 1% better at:

: ....
: ....
: ....

As I prepare to close my eyes
I am grateful for:

: ....
: ....
: ....

pen/pencil down
lights out
3 deep breaths

Only **97** days to go ➡ ➡ ➡ ➡

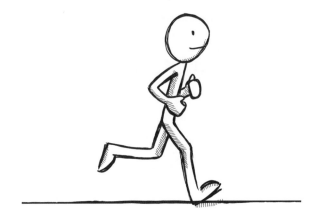

40 mins easy run

NOTES:

Location: ....
Weather: ....
Time start: _ _ /_ _ am/pm
Time finish: _ _ /_ _ am/pm

DAY 23: ☐ **DANG AND DONE iT!**

tick box

Woke up at: _ _ /_ _ am/pm
In bed now: _ _ /_ _ am/pm

Today I ate: OK ☐ WELL ☐ AWESOME ☐
My water intake was: OK ☐ GOOD ☐ AWESOME ☐
As a human I was: KIND ☐ THOUGHTFUL ☐ PRESENT ☐

Tomorrow I aim to be 1% better at:

: ....
: ....
: ....

As I prepare to close my eyes
I am grateful for:

: ....
: ....
: ....

pen/pencil down
lights out
3 deep breaths

Only **96** days to go ➡ ➡ ➡

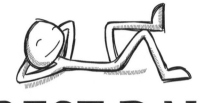

REST DAY

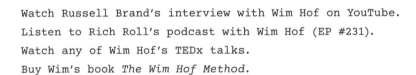

COLD SHOWER TIME!!

You HAVE to start COLD-SHOWERING!!

A COLD SHOWER FIRST THING IN THE MORNING
IS SO UNBELIEVABLY GOOD FOR YOU!!

IF YOU DON'T BELIEVE ME:

Watch Russell Brand's interview with Wim Hof on YouTube.
Listen to Rich Roll's podcast with Wim Hof (EP #231).
Watch any of Wim Hof's TEDx talks.
Buy Wim's book *The Wim Hof Method*.

CAN YOU SPOT A THEME HERE?

Wim is *the* Man. He is *the* Cold Water Therapy Guru.

IT'S TIME TO JUMP IN THE SHOWER
AND FEEL THE BURN - OF THE COLD!!

YOUR ENERGY LEVELS AND ALL-ROUND
WELLNESS ARE ABOUT TO CHANGE FOREVER!!

DAY 24: 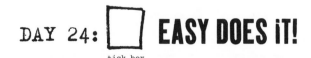 **EASY DOES iT!**

tick box

```
Week 4: Wednesday: _ _ /_ _ /_ _
```

Woke up at: _ _ /_ _ am/pm
In bed now: _ _ /_ _ am/pm

Today I ate: **OK** ☐ WELL ☐ AWESOME ☐
My water intake was: **OK** ☐ GOOD ☐ AWESOME ☐
As a human I was: KIND ☐ THOUGHTFUL ☐ PRESENT ☐

Tomorrow I aim to be 1% better at:

: ....
: ....
: ....

As I prepare to close my eyes
I am grateful for:

: ....
: ....
: ....

pen/pencil down
lights out
3 deep breaths

Only **95** days to go ➧➧➧➧

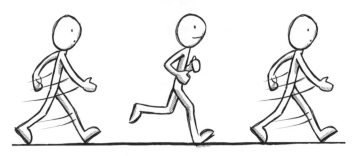

5 mins brisk walk/
45 mins easy run/
5 mins brisk walk
= **55 mins total**

NOTES:

Location: ....

Weather: ....

Time start: _ _ /_ _ am/pm

Time finish: _ _ /_ _ am/pm

DAY 25: ☐ **WORD UP!**

tick box

```
Week 4: Thursday: _ _ /_ _ /_ _
```

Woke up at: _ _ /_ _ am/pm
In bed now: _ _ /_ _ am/pm

Today I ate: OK ☐ WELL ☐ AWESOME ☐
My water intake was: OK ☐ GOOD ☐ AWESOME ☐
As a human I was: KIND ☐ THOUGHTFUL ☐ PRESENT ☐

Tomorrow I aim to be 1% better at:

: ....
: ....
: ....

As I prepare to close my eyes
I am grateful for:

: ....
: ....
: ....

pen/pencil down
lights out
3 deep breaths

Only **94** days to go ➡➡➡➡

DAY
26

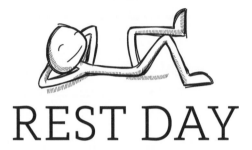

REST DAY

IN CASE YOU HAVE STILL NOT COLD-SHOWERED ...

YOU HAVE TO!!

**Make today the day you finally become a proud member
of the worldwide (MILDLY UNHINGED) cold shower club.**

Take the oath. Say after me:

'From this moment on, I do solemnly swear, to take a cold
shower every morning, every day, for the rest of my life.'

- Begin with a few seconds a day, for the first week or two.
- Aim to build up to 30 seconds within a fortnight.
- From there, two minutes is the ultimate target.

BUT ANYTHING IS BETTER THAN NOTHING!

I have been cold-showering every morning now for over two years.
I can honestly say that, except for two nights when I was admitted
to hospital for a medical emergency. I have never ever missed
a single day, or ever felt better in my life. During this time,
my hay fever (which I'd had since I was a teenager) has also
completely disappeared.

GO FOR IT!!

DAY 26: ☐ **YEE HA!**

tick box

Week 4: Friday: _ _ /_ _ /_ _

Woke up at: _ _ /_ _ am/pm
In bed now: _ _ /_ _ am/pm

Today I ate: OK ☐ WELL ☐ AWESOME ☐
My water intake was: OK ☐ GOOD ☐ AWESOME ☐
As a human I was: KIND ☐ THOUGHTFUL ☐ PRESENT ☐

Tomorrow I aim to be 1% better at:

: ....
: ....
: ....

As I prepare to close my eyes
I am grateful for:

: ....
: ....
: ....

pen/pencil down
lights out
3 deep breaths

Only **93** days to go ➡➡➡➡

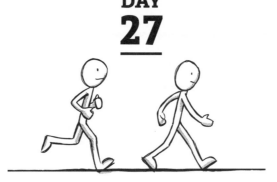

40 mins easy run/walk

EASY. EASY. EASY. WE LOVE SATURDAYS!!

BRING ON THE COCONUT FLAT WHITE!

Take a few moments this morning to meditate on the cause you have chosen to run for, who you will be helping and how much they will appreciate all your effort, hard work, kindness and consideration.

If you are yet to engage with a cause or charity, make a commitment to yourself to do it this week. Maybe even this afternoon or sometime tomorrow, while you're more relaxed, have more time, energy and extra headspace to choose the cause that inspires and speaks to you most.

From now on during your walk/run training, if you feel like you want to start jogging/shuffling/running sooner and for longer, if it feels right and you feel strong - GO FOR IT!

You have nothing to fear and everything to gain.

Location: ....

Weather: ....

Time start: _ _ /_ _ am/pm

Time finish: _ _ /_ _ am/pm

DAY 27:

tick box

NAiLED!

Woke up at: _ _ /_ _ am/pm
In bed now: _ _ /_ _ am/pm

Today I ate: OK ☐ WELL ☐ AWESOME ☐
My water intake was: OK ☐ GOOD ☐ AWESOME ☐
As a human I was: KIND ☐ THOUGHTFUL ☐ PRESENT ☐

Tomorrow I aim to be 1% better at:

: ....
: ....
: ....

As I prepare to close my eyes
I am grateful for:

: ....
: ....
: ....

pen/pencil down
lights out
3 deep breaths

Only **92** days to go ➡ ➡ ➡

LONG **DAY 28** RUN

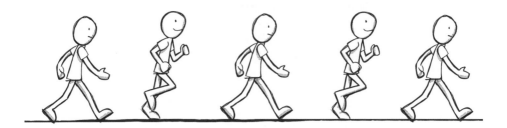

10 mins walk/30 mins jog/ 10 mins walk/30 mins jog/ 10 mins walk = **90 mins total**

YOUR FOURTH LONG-RUN DAY!

LONG RUN NUMBER 4

Location: ....

Weather: ....

Time start: _ _ / _ _ am/pm

Time finish: _ _ / _ _ am/pm

Mood before: ....

Mood after: ....

WRITE DOWN FIVE WORDS TO DESCRIBE YOUR DAY TODAY:

1. ....
2. ....
3. ....

4. ....
5. ....

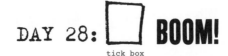

DAY 28: ☐ **BOOM!**

tick box

Week 4: Sunday: _ _ /_ _ /_ _

NIGHTY NIGHT WEEK 4

Woke up at: _ _ /_ _ am/pm
In bed now: _ _ /_ _ am/pm

This week my diet has been OK ☐ PRETTY GOOD ☐ AWESOME ☐

This week I have slept OK ☐ WELL ☐ AMAZINGLY ☐

This week my training has gone OK ☐ WELL ☐ AWESOMELY ☐

Going into WEEK 5 I will:

1. Make a commitment to take a brief cold shower every day,
first thing YES ☐ NO ☐

2. Watch/listen to at least one Wim Hof cold shower
masterclass online YES ☐ NO ☐

3. Gently begin to reduce the walking aspect of my
training YES ☐ NO ☐

As I prepare to close my eyes at the end of WEEK 4, I am grateful for:

1 ....

2 ....

3 ....

Next week in my training I aim to be 1 PER CENT better at:

....

pen/pencil down, lights out, 3 deep breaths

WEEK 4 OFFiCiALLY SMASHED ☐

tick box

Week 5

FEELiN' GOOD!

AT A GLANCE:

Tues: 30 mins easy run

Thurs: 30 mins easy run

Sat: 40 mins easy run/walk

Sun: 25 mins easy run,
2 mins walk, 25 mins easy run

TOTAL TRAINING TIME:
2 hrs 32 mins

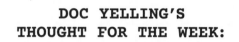

DOC YELLING'S
THOUGHT FOR THE WEEK:

The honeymoon period is now officially over.
Welcome to the second phase of your marathon
training plan. You have smashed Phase 1. How cool
is that? Time now to hunker down and launch yourself
towards the halfway point. This week the runs
are continuous but a little shorter in duration.
Bank them and boost your confidence!!!

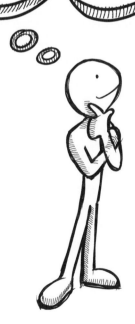

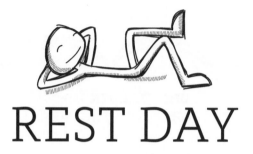

REST DAY

DON'T

THINK

ABOUT RUNNING

OR

ANYTHING

TO

DO

WITH

RUNNING

AT

ALL

(SEE YOU TOMORROW)

DAY 29: ☐ **HOOPLA!**

tick box

Week 5: Monday: _ _ /_ _ /_ _

Woke up at: _ _ /_ _ am/pm
In bed now: _ _ /_ _ am/pm

Today I ate: **OK** ☐ WELL ☐ AWESOME ☐
My water intake was: **OK** ☐ GOOD ☐ AWESOME ☐
As a human I was: KIND ☐ THOUGHTFUL ☐ PRESENT ☐

Tomorrow I aim to be 1% better at:

: ....
: ....
: ....

As I prepare to close my eyes
I am grateful for:

: ....
: ....
: ....

pen/pencil down
lights out
3 deep breaths

Only **90** days to go ➡➡➡➡

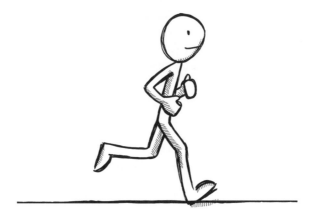

30 mins easy run

NOTES:

Location: ....

Weather: ....

Time start: _ _ /_ _ am/pm

Time finish: _ _ /_ _ am/pm

DAY 30: ☐ **CHAMPiON!**

tick box

Week 5: Tuesday: _ _ /_ _ /_ _

Woke up at: _ _ /_ _ am/pm
In bed now: _ _ /_ _ am/pm

Today I ate: OK ☐ WELL ☐ AWESOME ☐
My water intake was: OK ☐ GOOD ☐ AWESOME ☐
As a human I was: KIND ☐ THOUGHTFUL ☐ PRESENT ☐

Tomorrow I aim to be 1% better at:

: ....
: ....
: ....

As I prepare to close my eyes
I am grateful for:

: ....
: ....
: ....

pen/pencil down
lights out
3 deep breaths

Only **89** days to go ➡➡➡

DAY
31

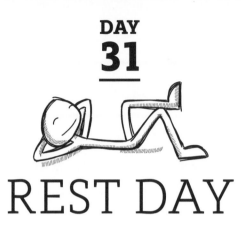

REST DAY

IT'S TIME TO TALK ABOUT WATER AGAIN, BUT THIS TIME HOW MUCH WE
NEED TO CONSUME.

IT'S NOT ONLY ABOUT HOW MUCH WATER WE DRINK.
IT'S ALSO ABOUT HOW MUCH WATER WE EAT.

WE HUMANS CAN BE PRETTY STUPID AT THE BEST OF TIMES.

But when it comes to our water intake, we excel. The general
picture is that, on average, we require between 2 to 3 litres of
water a day depending on our size, the weather, how much energy
we have been expending and, as in my case, whether we are prone
to things such as kidney stones. Three of which I fell victim
to while writing this book!! OUCH!!

BUT BUT BUT BUT BUT BUT BUT BUT BUT BUT BUT BUUUUT!!

2-3 litres in TOTAL, from both what we drink AND OUR FOOD!

As we are roughly 70 per cent water ourselves,
a good rule of thumb is to try to eat meals
that also consist of at least 70 per cent water.

DAY 31:

☐

tick box

FRESH FRUIT = 90 PER CENT WATER.
FRESH VEGETABLES = 70 PER CENT WATER.

SPLASH
BOOM!

DRINK PLENTY OF WATER.
BUT REMEMBER TO EAT LOTS OF WATER TOO!

It's not rocket science, BUT IT IS SCIENCE. Wise up, people!!

Week 5: Wednesday: _ _ /_ _ /_ _

Woke up at: _ _ /_ _ am/pm
In bed now: _ _ /_ _ am/pm

Today I ate: OK ☐ WELL ☐ AWESOME ☐
My water intake was: OK ☐ GOOD ☐ AWESOME ☐
As a human I was: KIND ☐ THOUGHTFUL ☐ PRESENT ☐

Tomorrow I aim to be 1% better at:

: ....
: ....
: ....

As I prepare to close my eyes
I am grateful for:

: ....
: ....
: ....

pen/pencil down
lights out
3 deep breaths

Only **88** days to go ➡➡➡

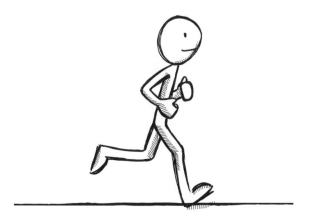

30 mins easy run

NOTES:

Location: ....

Weather: ....

Time start: _ _ /_ _ am/pm

Time finish: _ _ /_ _ am/pm

DAY 32: ☐ **JOB DONE!**

tick box

Week 5: Thursday: _ _ /_ _ /_ _

Woke up at: _ _ /_ _ am/pm
In bed now: _ _ /_ _ am/pm

Today I ate: OK ☐ WELL ☐ AWESOME ☐
My water intake was: OK ☐ GOOD ☐ AWESOME ☐
As a human I was: KIND ☐ THOUGHTFUL ☐ PRESENT ☐

Tomorrow I aim to be 1% better at:

: ....
: ....
: ....

As I prepare to close my eyes
I am grateful for:

: ....
: ....
: ....

pen/pencil down
lights out
3 deep breaths

Only **87** days to go ➡ ➡ ➡ ➡

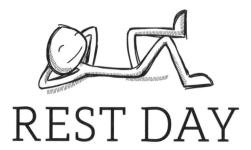

REST DAY

BONUS TOP 5 WATER FUN FACTS

1. The global bottled water industry's projected turnover for 2022 is $319.8 billion!!

2. In the UK, over 7 billion single-use plastic water bottles are bought and discarded every year.

3. Some bottled water companies source their water from THE TAP!!

4. UK domestic water standards (TAP WATER!!) are among the highest in the world.

5. Simply drinking a glass of good old UK tap water while reading can help transport nutrients around your body, aid the excretion of waste products, and improve your focus and concentration within minutes.

INVEST IN A DECENT WATER BOTTLE.
GIVE PRAISE FOR YOUR TAP AND UK WATER
STANDARDS. SAVE A SMALL FORTUNE WHILE
HELPING SAVE THE PLANET.

DAY 33: **ALRiGHT!** ☐ **CHEERS!**

tick box

Week 5: Friday: _ _ /_ _ /_ _

Woke up at: _ _ /_ _ am/pm
In bed now: _ _ /_ _ am/pm

Today I ate: OK ☐ WELL ☐ AWESOME ☐
My water intake was: OK ☐ GOOD ☐ AWESOME ☐
As a human I was: KIND ☐ THOUGHTFUL ☐ PRESENT ☐

Tomorrow I aim to be 1% better at:

: ....
: ....
: ....

As I prepare to close my eyes
I am grateful for:

: ....
: ....
: ....

pen/pencil down
lights out
3 deep breaths

Only **86** days to go ➡ ➡ ➡ ➡

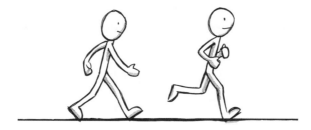

40 mins easy walk/run

HAPPY SATURDAY, MY SATURDAY
EASY WALK/RUN, FRIENDS!

ONE MORE WATER HACK. JUST FOR LUCK.

Always keep a small bottle of frozen water in the freezer. This
can double as a highly effective, supercooled, mini muscle-roller.

As your mile count begins to steadily creep up over the next few
weeks, treat the soles of your feet to a cheeky little chilled
roll, every now and again.

This can work wonders to help boost recovery, as well as helping
stave off any early signs of the dreaded plantar fasciitis.

THIS IS ALL BECAUSE YOU ARE SLOWLY BUT
SURELY BECOMING A BONA FIDE ENDURANCE ATHLETE.
YOU ROCK - BIG TIME!!

Location: ....

Weather: ....

Time start: _ _ /_ _ am/pm

Time finish: _ _ /_ _ am/pm

DAY 34:

tick box

SMASHED –
OOH YAH!

Woke up at: _ _ /_ _ am/pm
In bed now: _ _ /_ _ am/pm

Today I ate: **OK** ☐ WELL ☐ AWESOME ☐
My water intake was: **OK** ☐ GOOD ☐ AWESOME ☐
As a human I was: KIND ☐ THOUGHTFUL ☐ PRESENT ☐

Tomorrow I aim to be 1% better at:

: ....
: ....
: ....

As I prepare to close my eyes
I am grateful for:

: ....
: ....
: ....

pen/pencil down
lights out
3 deep breaths

Only **85** days to go ➡➡➡➡

LONG **DAY** **35** RUN

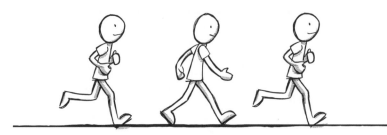

25 mins easy run/
2 mins walk/25 mins easy run
= **52 mins total**

YOUR FIFTH LONG-RUN DAY
(ALTHOUGH NOT ACTUALLY THAT LONG!)

LONG RUN NUMBER 5

Location: ....

Weather: ....

Time start: _ _ /_ _ am/pm

Time finish: _ _ /_ _ am/pm

Mood before: ....

Mood after: ....

WRITE DOWN FIVE WORDS TO DESCRIBE YOUR DAY TODAY:

1. ....
2. ....
3. ....

4. ....
5. ....

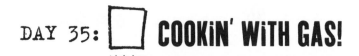

DAY 35: COOKiN' WiTH GAS!

tick box

Week 5: Sunday: _ _ /_ _ /_ _

NIGHTY NIGHT WEEK 5

Woke up at: _ _ /_ _ am/pm
In bed now: _ _ /_ _ am/pm

This week my diet has been OK ☐ PRETTY GOOD ☐ AWESOME ☐

This week I have slept OK ☐ WELL ☐ AMAZINGLY ☐

This week my training has gone OK ☐ WELL ☐ AWESOMELY ☐

Going into WEEK 6 I will:

1. Enter a whole new water world of hydration and food YES ☐ NO ☐

2. Deploy a refillable water bottle YES ☐ NO ☐

3. Enjoy an endless supply of FREE HEALTHY TAP WATER YES ☐ NO ☐

As I prepare to close my eyes at the
end of WEEK 5, I am grateful for:

1 ....

2 ....

3 ....

Next week in my training I aim to be
1 PER CENT better at:

....

pen/pencil down, lights out, 3 deep breaths

WEEK 5 OFFICIALLY SMASHED ☐

tick box

Week 6

LOOKiN' GOOD!

AT A GLANCE:

Tues: 40 mins easy run

Thurs: 10 mins easy run/
(1 min tempo run, 2 mins walk)
x 8/10 mins easy jog = 44 mins total

Sat: 50 mins walk/run

Sun: (20 mins easy run, 5 mins brisk walk) x 4
= 1 hr 40 mins total

TOTAL TRAINING TIME: 3 hrs 54 mins

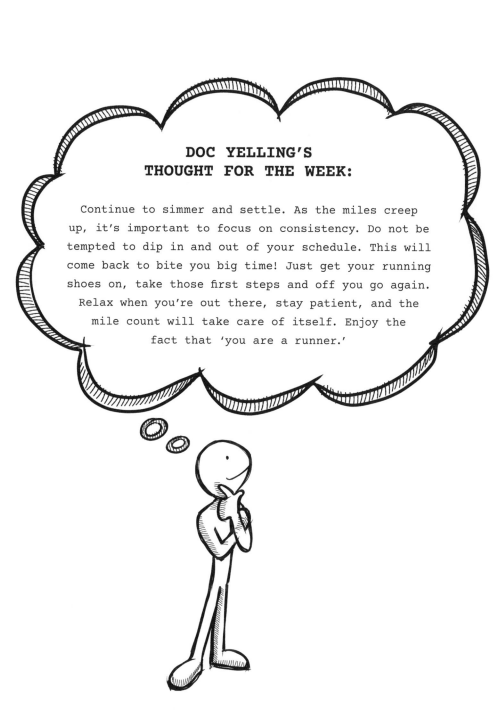

**DOC YELLING'S
THOUGHT FOR THE WEEK:**

Continue to simmer and settle. As the miles creep
up, it's important to focus on consistency. Do not be
tempted to dip in and out of your schedule. This will
come back to bite you big time! Just get your running
shoes on, take those first steps and off you go again.
Relax when you're out there, stay patient, and the
mile count will take care of itself. Enjoy the
fact that 'you are a runner.'

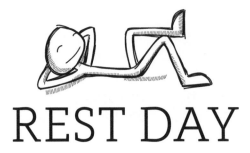

REST DAY

DON'T

THINK

ABOUT RUNNING

OR

ANYTHING

TO

DO

WITH

RUNNING

AT

ALL

(SEE YOU TOMORROW)

DAY 36: ⬜ **HURRAH!**

tick box

```
Week 6: Monday: _ _ /_ _ /_ _
```

Woke up at: _ _ /_ _ am/pm
In bed now: _ _ /_ _ am/pm

Today I ate: OK ☐ WELL ☐ AWESOME ☐
My water intake was: OK ☐ GOOD ☐ AWESOME ☐
As a human I was: KIND ☐ THOUGHTFUL ☐ PRESENT ☐

Tomorrow I aim to be 1% better at:

: ....
: ....
: ....

As I prepare to close my eyes
I am grateful for:

: ....
: ....
: ....

pen/pencil down
lights out
3 deep breaths

Only **83** days to go ➡ ➡ ➡

DAY
37

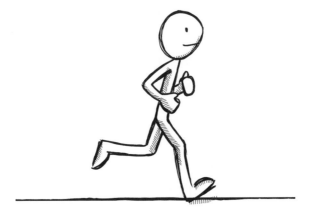

40 mins easy run

NOTES:

```
Location:    .........................
Weather:     .........................
Time start:  _ _ /_ _ am/pm
Time finish: _ _ /_ _ am/pm
```

DAY 37: [ ] **SORTED!**

tick box

```
Week 6: Tuesday: _ _ /_ _ /_ _
```

Woke up at: _ _ /_ _ am/pm
In bed now: _ _ /_ _ am/pm

Today I ate: OK ☐ WELL ☐ AWESOME ☐
My water intake was: OK ☐ GOOD ☐ AWESOME ☐
As a human I was: KIND ☐ THOUGHTFUL ☐ PRESENT ☐

Tomorrow I aim to be 1% better at:

: ....
: ....
: ....

As I prepare to close my eyes
I am grateful for:

: ....
: ....
: ....

pen/pencil down
lights out
3 deep breaths

Only **82** days to go ➡ ➡ ➡ ➡

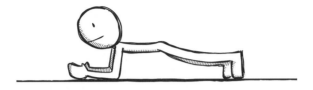

Rest Day/X-Train Day!!

YES, THAT'S RIGHT. FROM NOW ON, REST DAYS CAN ALSO DOUBLE AS CROSS-TRAINING DAYS, BUT DON'T PANIC - IT'S NOWHERE NEAR AS DRAMATIC AS IT SOUNDS.

IT'S TIME TO SAY THANK YOU TO YOUR LEGS!

This next little addition to your routine is like giving them a new superpower. More strength, more stamina, more race-day resolve and resilience.

Any type of light cross-training will do this. My cross-training of choice is based on 3 simple YouTube workouts that I've discovered over the last couple of years:

1. '7-MINUTE WORKOUT WITH INGER HOUGHTON'
2. '5-MINUTE BUTT AND THIGH WORKOUT WITH KELLY'
3. '10-MINUTE FAT-BURNING ROUTINE WITH ROWAN ROW'

The added benefits of any/all of the above SUPER QUICK workouts contributing to your confidence, fitness and positive mindset going into race-day are priceless.

WHY WOULD YOU NOT DO THIS??

DAY 38: **CROSSED AND TRAiNED!**

tick box

Week 6: Wednesday: _ _ /_ _ /_ _

Woke up at: _ _ /_ _ am/pm
In bed now: _ _ /_ _ am/pm

Today I ate: OK ☐ WELL ☐ AWESOME ☐
My water intake was: OK ☐ GOOD ☐ AWESOME ☐
As a human I was: KIND ☐ THOUGHTFUL ☐ PRESENT ☐

Tomorrow I aim to be 1% better at:

: ....
: ....
: ....

As I prepare to close my eyes
I am grateful for:

: ....
: ....
: ....

pen/pencil down
lights out
3 deep breaths

Only **81** days to go ➡ ➡ ➡ ➡

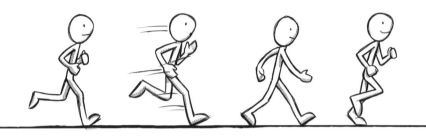

10 mins easy run/
(1 min tempo run, 2 mins walk)
x 8/10 mins easy jog
= **44 mins total**

NOTES:

```
Location: ...........................
Weather: ...........................
Time start: _ _ /_ _ am/pm
Time finish: _ _ /_ _ am/pm
```

DAY 39: ☐ **OKEY DOKEY!**

tick box

Week 6: Thursday: _ _ /_ _ /_ _

Woke up at: _ _ /_ _ am/pm
In bed now: _ _ /_ _ am/pm

Today I ate: OK ☐ WELL ☐ AWESOME ☐
My water intake was: OK ☐ GOOD ☐ AWESOME ☐
As a human I was: KIND ☐ THOUGHTFUL ☐ PRESENT ☐

Tomorrow I aim to be 1% better at:

: ....
: ....
: ....

As I prepare to close my eyes
I am grateful for:

: ....
: ....
: ....

pen/pencil down
lights out
3 deep breaths

Only **80** days to go ➡➡➡➡

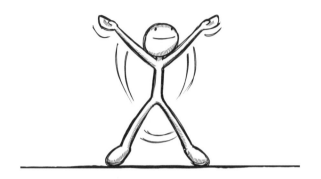

Rest Day/X-Train Day

BEST FRIDAY FUN THOUGHT OF ALL TIME:

HOW ABOUT BOOKING A TABLE AT A PUB/CURRY HOUSE/ITALIAN/CHINESE FOR A POST-RACE CELEBRATION DINNER WITH FRIENDS AND FAMILY?

F.W.I.W.: After each of my London marathons, I've met up with fellow runners, friends and family at my favourite pub in Primrose Hill in North London for pints, pizza and red wine. It's in my top 3 favourite nights of the year.

Once you have made your decision, **STICK IT IN THE DIARY. BOOM! THE VICTORY DINNER!! IT'S GOING TO HAPPEN!!**

(pssst ... You might even want to consider booking the Monday off work so you can really push the boat out!!)

DAY 40: **ABRA-KE-PUB-RA!**

tick box

```
Week 6: Friday: _ _ /_ _ /_ _
```

Woke up at: _ _ /_ _ am/pm
In bed now: _ _ /_ _ am/pm

Today I ate: OK ☐ WELL ☐ AWESOME ☐

My water intake was: OK ☐ GOOD ☐ AWESOME ☐

As a human I was: KIND ☐ THOUGHTFUL ☐ PRESENT ☐

Tomorrow I aim to be 1% better at:

: ....
: ....
: ....

**As I prepare to close my eyes
I am grateful for:**

: ....
: ....
: ....

pen/pencil down
lights out
3 deep breaths

Only **79** days to go ➡ ➡ ➡

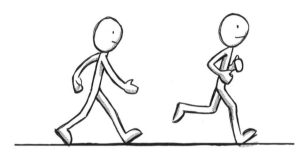

50 mins walk/run

ANOTHER SATURDAY, ANOTHER CHEEKY PRE-RUN COCONUT FLAT WHITE!

I love the early Saturday morning coffee line of like-minded runners/cyclists/walkers fuelling up for another outing. The infectious chatter, energy and positive vibes really help fire me up both psychologically and spiritually for another fulfilling weekend of training.

Being around your tribe, people who are on the same wavelength as you, is truly inspiring and reassuring. It also serves as an invaluable reminder that in all walks of life, achieving what you want is 90 per cent showing up, 10 per cent everything else.

WELL, STARTED IS HALF DONE!!

Location: ....

Weather: ....

Time start: _ _ /_ _ am/pm

Time finish: _ _ /_ _ am/pm

DAY 41:
TOTALLY
DONE!

tick box

Woke up at: _ _ /_ _ am/pm
In bed now: _ _ /_ _ am/pm

Today I ate: OK ☐ WELL ☐ AWESOME ☐
My water intake was: OK ☐ GOOD ☐ AWESOME ☐
As a human I was: KIND ☐ THOUGHTFUL ☐ PRESENT ☐

Tomorrow I aim to be 1% better at:

: ....
: ....
: ....

As I prepare to close my eyes
I am grateful for:

: ....
: ....
: ....

pen/pencil down
lights out
3 deep breaths

Only **78** days to go ➡ ➡ ➡ ➡

LONG **DAY 42** RUN

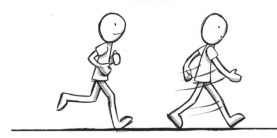

(20 mins easy run, 5 mins brisk walk) x 4
= 1 hr 40 mins total
Or distance goal: 6 to 8 miles

YOUR SIXTH LONG-RUN DAY!

LONG RUN NUMBER 6

Location: ....

Weather: ....

Time start: _ _ /_ _ am/pm

Time finish: _ _ /_ _ am/pm

Mood before: ....

Mood after: ....

WRITE DOWN FIVE WORDS TO DESCRIBE YOUR DAY TODAY:

1. ....
2. ....
3. ....

4. ....
5. ....

DAY 42: ☐ **GOOD EFFORT!**

tick box

Week 6: Sunday: _ _ /_ _ /_ _

NIGHTY NIGHT WEEK 6

Woke up at: _ _ /_ _ am/pm
In bed now: _ _ /_ _ am/pm

This week my diet has been OK ☐ PRETTY GOOD ☐ AWESOME ☐
This week I have slept OK ☐ WELL ☐ AMAZINGLY ☐
This week my training has gone OK ☐ WELL ☐ AWESOMELY ☐

Going into WEEK 7 I will:

1. Make cross-training part of my marathon plan YES ☐ NO ☐
2. Book a post-marathon-celebration night out YES ☐ NO ☐
3. Spend time around my running/fitness tribe/hangout YES ☐ NO ☐

As I prepare to close my eyes at the
end of WEEK 6, I am grateful for:

1 ....
2 ....
3 ....

Next week in my training I aim to be
1 PER CENT better at:

....

pen/pencil down, lights out, 3 deep breaths

WEEK 6 OFFICIALLY SMASHED ☐

tick box

Week 7

ON THE GAS!

AT A GLANCE:

Tues: 40 mins easy run

Thurs: 10 mins easy jog/
(1 min 30 secs tempo run, 2 mins walk/jog)
x 8/10 mins easy jog = 48 mins total

Sat: 50 mins easy walk/run

Sun: (30 mins run, 5 mins brisk walk) x 3
= 1 hr 45 mins total

TOTAL TRAINING TIME = 4 hrs

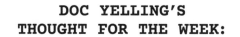

DOC YELLING'S
THOUGHT FOR THE WEEK:

This is where the foundations of the last 6 weeks truly
start to make a difference. You're layering up, your body
is learning to tolerate the miles that are yet to come.
Include some mixed-pace running to boost your fitness
and stay stronger for longer. When tempo running,
don't go big too early. Gradually increase your effort,
lengthen your stride, increase your cadence.
But staying SMOOTH is the key!

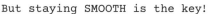

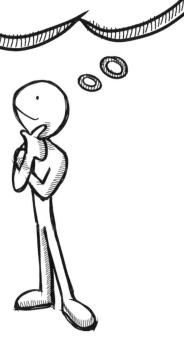

DAY
43

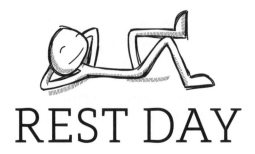

REST DAY

DON'T

THINK

ABOUT RUNNING

OR

ANYTHING

TO

DO

WITH

RUNNING

AT

ALL

(SEE YOU TOMORROW)

DAY 43: **HOLY MOLY!**

tick box

Woke up at: _ _ /_ _ am/pm
In bed now: _ _ /_ _ am/pm

Today I ate: OK ☐ WELL ☐ AWESOME ☐
My water intake was: OK ☐ GOOD ☐ AWESOME ☐
As a human I was: KIND ☐ THOUGHTFUL ☐ PRESENT ☐

Tomorrow I aim to be 1% better at:

: ....
: ....
: ....

As I prepare to close my eyes
I am grateful for:

: ....
: ....
: ....

pen/pencil down
lights out
3 deep breaths

Only **76** days to go ➡➡➡➡

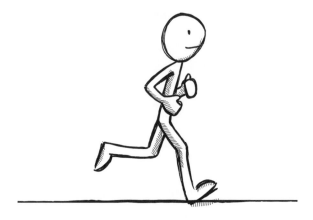

40 mins easy run

NOTES:

Location: ....

Weather: ....

Time start: _ _ /_ _ am/pm

Time finish: _ _ /_ _ am/pm

DAY 44: ☐ ON iT!

tick box

```
Week 7: Tuesday: _ _ /_ _ /_ _
```

Woke up at: _ _ /_ _ am/pm
In bed now: _ _ /_ _ am/pm

Today I ate: OK ☐ WELL ☐ AWESOME ☐
My water intake was: OK ☐ GOOD ☐ AWESOME ☐
As a human I was: KIND ☐ THOUGHTFUL ☐ PRESENT ☐

Tomorrow I aim to be 1% better at:

: ....
: ....
: ....

As I prepare to close my eyes
I am grateful for:

: ....
: ....
: ....

pen/pencil down
lights out
3 deep breaths

Only 75 days to go ➡➡➡

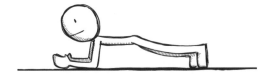

Rest Day/X-Train Day

OKAY. IT'S THAT TIME, MY FRIENDS. TIME TO START THINKING ABOUT WHAT TIME TO GO FOR.

That said, it's not all urgent - yet - but it is really important. You may think: 'Isn't it enough that I have committed to completing a marathon?' To which the answer is 100 per cent yes. However, having a time in mind, as soon into your training as feels comfortable, will help in so many ways.

To compute yours, merely begin to quietly consider what a realistic, sustainable pace might begin to feel like as you're out there running, especially on long-run days. Perhaps you're already beginning to sense what that time might be.

If you do have a time/pace already in mind, fantastic! But don't worry if you haven't. Listen to your body and it will let you know whereabouts you need to be between now and race day. And remember, nothing is written in stone at any point. Whatever target pace you go for initially is an entirely reversible decision

F.W.I.W.: I consulted a pal of similar age and fitness who had run his first marathon a year before mine. He said his goal was to finish in under 5 hours, which is approximately an 11 minutes 30 seconds a mile pace. So that's what I went for, and that's what happened.

DAY 45: 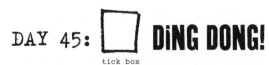 **DING DONG!**

tick box

Week 7: Wednesday: _ _ /_ _ /_ _

Woke up at: _ _ /_ _ am/pm
In bed now: _ _ /_ _ am/pm

Today I ate: OK ☐ WELL ☐ AWESOME ☐
My water intake was: OK ☐ GOOD ☐ AWESOME ☐
As a human I was: KIND ☐ THOUGHTFUL ☐ PRESENT ☐

Tomorrow I aim to be 1% better at:

: ....
: ....
: ....

As I prepare to close my eyes
I am grateful for:

: ....
: ....
: ....

pen/pencil down
lights out
3 deep breaths

Only 74 days to go ➡ ➡ ➡ ➡

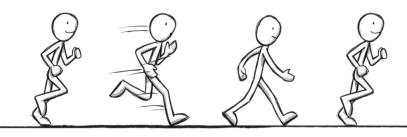

10 mins easy jog/
(1 min 30 secs tempo run,
2 mins walk/jog)
x 8/10 mins easy jog
= **48 mins total**

NOTES:

Location: ....
Weather: ....
Time start: _ _ /_ _ am/pm
Time finish: _ _ /_ _ am/pm

DAY 46: **NEVER iN DOUBT!**

tick box

Week 7: Thursday: _ _ /_ _ /_ _

Woke up at: _ _ /_ _ am/pm
In bed now: _ _ /_ _ am/pm

Today I ate: OK ☐ WELL ☐ AWESOME ☐
My water intake was: OK ☐ GOOD ☐ AWESOME ☐
As a human I was: KIND ☐ THOUGHTFUL ☐ PRESENT ☐

Tomorrow I aim to be 1% better at:

: ....
: ....
: ....

As I prepare to close my eyes
I am grateful for:

: ....
: ....
: ....

pen/pencil down
lights out
3 deep breaths

Only **73** days to go ➡➡➡➡

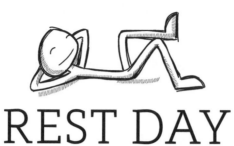

REST DAY

I know it's only been 48 hours but I bet you've been thinking about little else other than your target marathon pace time. Once the target pace time seed has been posed, it's difficult to focus on anything else in life until you have made an initial decision.

Why not make a rough guess now ahead of this weekend's long run and then give it a go and see how it works out?

As I've already mentioned, I plumped for sub-5 hours (at almost precisely this point in my training!). I then consulted a 'minutes per mile' table online, which informed me that I would therefore need to cover each mile in 11 minutes 35 seconds or better. Thus, I began to tailor my training to that end.

Without any doubt whatsoever, I can honestly tell you, this decision was the most empowering single moment of my whole training experience. Suddenly, everything became much clearer from that point. I knew what I wanted to do and how I wanted to do it. Just writing that now still makes the hairs stand up on the back of my neck.

And remember, I'm going through it all again with you this year, and guess what? I'm still aiming for sub-5. I'm still bricking myself. I'm still not sure I'll be able to pull it off and I'm still loving every second!! The perfect combination of excitement, anticipation, nervousness, uncertainty and commitment.

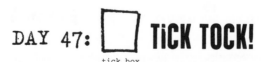

DAY 47: **TiCK TOCK!**

tick box

```
┌─────────────────────────────────────────────┐
│                                             │
│     Week 7: Friday: _ _ /_ _ /_ _           │
│                                             │
└─────────────────────────────────────────────┘
```

Woke up at: _ _ /_ _ am/pm
In bed now: _ _ /_ _ am/pm

Today I ate: OK ☐ WELL ☐ AWESOME ☐
My water intake was: OK ☐ GOOD ☐ AWESOME ☐
As a human I was: KIND ☐ THOUGHTFUL ☐ PRESENT ☐

Tomorrow I aim to be 1% better at:

: ....
: ....
: ....

As I prepare to close my eyes
I am grateful for:

: ....
: ....
: ....

pen/pencil down
lights out
3 deep breaths

Only **72** days to go ➤➤➤➤

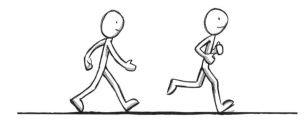

50 mins easy walk/run

DEAR BRAIN,

Things are beginning to get ever so slightly, wonderfully serious. I can feel it and I absolutely love it. But please help me to remind myself: training has to be PLAY FIRST and EVERYTHING ELSE SECOND. ALWAYS!!

We are not fighting wars or saving lives here. (Although many of us will be helping save lives depending on what causes we're running for. How cool is that?) I have simply made a commitment to myself, to do something that will reveal more of who I am today, to help me become more of who I want to be tomorrow.

NOTES:

Location: ....

Weather: ....

Time start: _ _ /_ _ am/pm

Time finish: _ _ /_ _ am/pm

DAY 48:

tick box

BA DA BiNG!

Woke up at: _ _ /_ _ am/pm
In bed now: _ _ /_ _ am/pm

Today I ate: OK ☐ WELL ☐ AWESOME ☐
My water intake was: OK ☐ GOOD ☐ AWESOME ☐
As a human I was: KIND ☐ THOUGHTFUL ☐ PRESENT ☐

Tomorrow I aim to be 1% better at:

: ....
: ....
: ....

As I prepare to close my eyes
I am grateful for:

: ....
: ....
: ....

pen/pencil down
lights out
3 deep breaths

Only 71 days to go ➡➡➡➡

LONG DAY **49** RUN

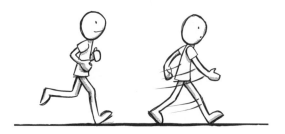

(30 mins run, 5 mins brisk walk) x 3
= 1 hr 45 mins total
Or distance goal: 8 to 10 miles

YOUR SEVENTH LONG-RUN DAY!

LONG RUN NUMBER 7

Location: ....

Weather: ....

Time start: _ _ /_ _ am/pm

Time finish: _ _ /_ _ am/pm

Mood before: ....

Mood after: ....

WRITE DOWN FIVE WORDS TO DESCRIBE YOUR DAY TODAY:

1. ....
2. ....
3. ....

4. ....
5. ....

DAY 49: ☐ EPiC!

tick box

Week 7: Sunday: _ _ /_ _ /_ _

NIGHTY NIGHT WEEK 7

Woke up at: _ _ /_ _ am/pm
In bed now: _ _ /_ _ am/pm

This week my diet has been OK ☐ PRETTY GOOD ☐ AWESOME ☐

This week I have slept OK ☐ WELL ☐ AMAZINGLY ☐

This week my training has gone OK ☐ WELL ☐ AWESOMELY ☐

Going into WEEK 8 I will:

1. Try to recognise my natural long-distance running pace YES ☐ NO ☐

2. Have a gut feel for my initial race pace YES ☐ NO ☐

3. Remember both can be adjusted at any point before race day YES ☐ NO ☐

As I prepare to close my eyes at the end of WEEK 7, I am grateful for:

1 ....

2 ....

3 ....

Next week in my training I aim to be 1 PER CENT better at:

....

pen/pencil down, lights out, 3 deep breaths

WEEK 7 OFFICIALLY SMASHED

tick box

Week 8

TURN UP THE HEAT!

AT A GLANCE:

Tues: 40 mins EASY RUN

Thurs: 50 mins JOG/TEMPO RUN/WALK

Sat: 60 mins WALK/RUN

Sun: 120 mins WALK/JOG

TOTAL TRAINING TIME: 4 hrs 30 mins

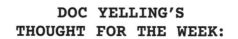

**DOC YELLING'S
THOUGHT FOR THE WEEK:**

As you approach halfway (HALFWAY!!! A-MAZE!!!),
start to think a bit more about fuelling and
hydration. When and what are you eating and drinking
around your long runs? Including the regulation of
comfort breaks! It's astounding how achievable these
can be once you begin to really dial in your
weekend food and drink schedule.

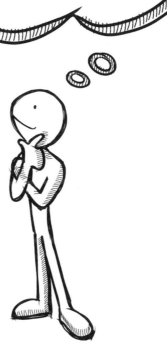

DAY
50

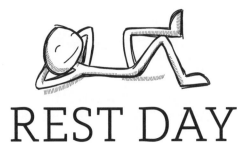

REST DAY

DON'T

THINK

ABOUT RUNNING

OR

ANYTHING

TO

DO

WITH

RUNNING

AT

ALL

(SEE YOU TOMORROW)

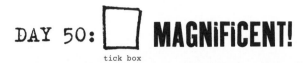

DAY 50: ☐ **MAGNiFiCENT!**

tick box

Woke up at: _ _ /_ _ am/pm
In bed now: _ _ /_ _ am/pm

Today I ate: OK ☐ WELL ☐ AWESOME ☐
My water intake was: OK ☐ GOOD ☐ AWESOME ☐
As a human I was: KIND ☐ THOUGHTFUL ☐ PRESENT ☐

Tomorrow I aim to be 1% better at:

: ....

: ....

: ....

As I prepare to close my eyes
I am grateful for:

: ....

: ....

: ....

pen/pencil down
lights out
3 deep breaths

Only **69** days to go ➡ ➡ ➡ ➡

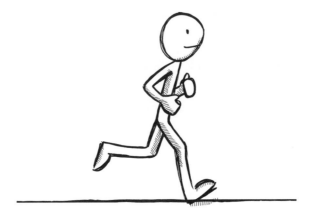

40 mins easy run

NOTES:

Location: ....

Weather: ....

Time start: _ _ /_ _ am/pm

Time finish: _ _ /_ _ am/pm

DAY 51: 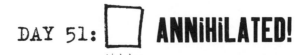 ANNiHiLATED!

tick box

Week 8: Tuesday: _ _ /_ _ /_ _

Woke up at: _ _ /_ _ am/pm
In bed now: _ _ /_ _ am/pm

Today I ate: OK ☐ WELL ☐ AWESOME ☐
My water intake was: OK ☐ GOOD ☐ AWESOME ☐
As a human I was: KIND ☐ THOUGHTFUL ☐ PRESENT ☐

Tomorrow I aim to be 1% better at:

: ....
: ....
: ....

As I prepare to close my eyes
I am grateful for:

: ....
: ....
: ....

pen/pencil down
lights out
3 deep breaths

Only **68** days to go ➡ ➡ ➡ ➡

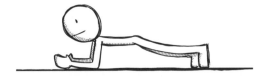

Rest Day/X-Train Day

DEAR BRAIN,

Have we ever considered meditation as an alternative energy source? Or even an alternative sauce?

F.W.I.W.: You don't have to believe in gravity for it to work. The same can be said of meditation. All I want to tell you is that since I started meditating (20 minutes in the morning and 20 minutes in the afternoon), I feel completely different. Maybe this is for another book, but meditation has profoundly changed my life for the better, even more than running.

That said, I don't think I would have arrived at meditation were it not for the rite of passage that is running. Stillness speaks volumes, it's who we really are. When you can access your inner stillness at will, you have all the power a human being needs.

I'll leave it there for now. I won't push it, save to say, don't worry about 'not being able to sit still in silence for more than a minute, let alone 20 minutes!' If you meditate correctly (which is with minimal effort and so much easier than you can possibly imagine), the time flies by. You don't have to take my word for it. Give it a go!

DAY 52: **MEDITATED!**

tick box

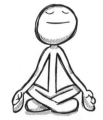

Week 8: Wednesday: _ _ /_ _ /_ _

Woke up at: _ _ /_ _ am/pm
In bed now: _ _ /_ _ am/pm

Today I ate: OK ☐ WELL ☐ AWESOME ☐
My water intake was: OK ☐ GOOD ☐ AWESOME ☐
As a human I was: KIND ☐ THOUGHTFUL ☐ PRESENT ☐

Tomorrow I aim to be 1% better at:

: ....
: ....
: ....

As I prepare to close my eyes
I am grateful for:

: ....
: ....
: ....

pen/pencil down
lights out
3 deep breaths

Only **67** days to go ➡ ➡ ➡ ➡

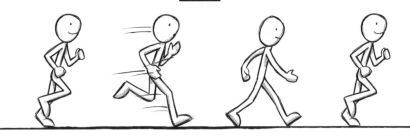

10 mins easy jog/
(2 mins tempo run,
2 mins walk/jog)
x 8/10 mins easy jog
= 52 mins total

NOTES:

Location: ....

Weather: ....

Time start: _ _ /_ _ am/pm

Time finish: _ _ /_ _ am/pm

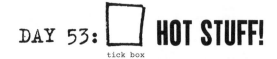

DAY 53: ☐ **HOT STUFF!**

tick box

Week 8: Thursday: _ _ /_ _ /_ _

Woke up at: _ _ /_ _ am/pm
In bed now: _ _ /_ _ am/pm

Today I ate: OK ☐ WELL ☐ AWESOME ☐
My water intake was: OK ☐ GOOD ☐ AWESOME ☐
As a human I was: KIND ☐ THOUGHTFUL ☐ PRESENT ☐

Tomorrow I aim to be 1% better at:

: ....
: ....
: ....

As I prepare to close my eyes
I am grateful for:

: ....
: ....
: ....

pen/pencil down
lights out
3 deep breaths

Only **66** days to go ➡ ➡ ➡ ➡

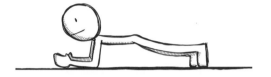

Rest Day/X-Train Day

FUN FRIDAY THOUGHT:

Are you missing a bit of weekend madness? Do you fancy a mid-marathon training, Saturday night blowout?

WELL, HOW ABOUT THIS FOR A CHEEKY TRAINING PLAN CURVE BALL!!

Why don't you treat yourself by changing one of your Sunday morning long runs to Saturday? Then take Sunday as the first rest day of the following week and move everything one day forward until your next long run.

No one's holding you to ransom here.

That said, don't go too crazy. You've already put in tons of heavy lifting, energy, focus and commitment. It would be madness to jeopardise all that effort for the sake of one too many cold drinks. But here we are, roughly halfway to the big day. One relaxed night out, after a long run, with a bit of reflection thrown in, isn't going to do any harm. Besides, you might be pleasantly surprised, once you give yourself permission to let off a bit of steam – shock, horror, you might not even want to.

It's amazing how quickly our bodies can change to craving what they need as opposed to what we want.

DAY 54: KABOOM!

tick box

Week 8: Friday: _ _ /_ _ /_ _

Woke up at: _ _ /_ _ am/pm
In bed now: _ _ /_ _ am/pm

Today I ate: OK ☐ WELL ☐ AWESOME ☐
My water intake was: OK ☐ GOOD ☐ AWESOME ☐
As a human I was: KIND ☐ THOUGHTFUL ☐ PRESENT ☐

Tomorrow I aim to be 1% better at:

: ....
: ....
: ....

As I prepare to close my eyes
I am grateful for:

: ....
: ....
: ....

pen/pencil down
lights out
3 deep breaths

Only **65** days to go ➡ ➡ ➡ ➡

DAY
55

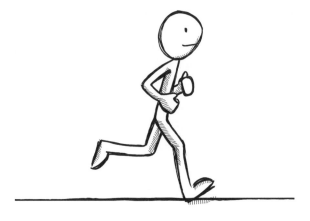

60 mins walk/run

NOTES:

```
Location: .........................
Weather: .........................
Time start: _ _ /_ _ am/pm
Time finish: _ _ /_ _ am/pm
```

DAY 55: ☐ **HEAR HEAR!**

tick box

```
Week 8: Saturday: _ _ /_ _ /_ _
```

Woke up at: _ _ /_ _ am/pm
In bed now: _ _ /_ _ am/pm

Today I ate: **OK** ☐ WELL ☐ AWESOME ☐
My water intake was: **OK** ☐ GOOD ☐ AWESOME ☐
As a human I was: KIND ☐ THOUGHTFUL ☐ PRESENT ☐

Tomorrow I aim to be 1% better at:

: ....
: ....
: ....

As I prepare to close my eyes
I am grateful for:

: ....
: ....
: ....

pen/pencil down
lights out
3 deep breaths

Only **64** days to go ➡ ➡ ➡ ➡

LONG **DAY 56** RUN

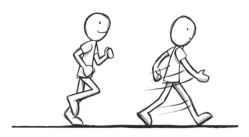

(25 mins jog,
5 mins brisk walk) x 4
= 2 hrs total
Or distance goal: 8 to 10 miles

YOUR EIGHTH LONG-RUN DAY!

LONG RUN NUMBER 8

Location: ....

Weather: ....

Time start: _ _ /_ _ am/pm

Time finish: _ _ /_ _ am/pm

Mood before: ....

Mood after: ....

WRITE DOWN FIVE WORDS TO DESCRIBE YOUR DAY TODAY:

1. ....
2. ....
3. ....

4. ....
5. ....

DAY 56: MONSTERED!

tick box

Week 8: Sunday: _ _ /_ _ /_ _

NIGHTY NIGHT WEEK 8

Woke up at: _ _ /_ _ am/pm
In bed now: _ _ /_ _ am/pm

This week my diet has been OK ☐ PRETTY GOOD ☐ AWESOME ☐

This week I have slept OK ☐ WELL ☐ AMAZINGLY ☐

This week my training has gone OK ☐ WELL ☐ AWESOMELY ☐

Going into WEEK 9 I will:

1. Try meditation for the first time YES ☐ NO ☐

2. Watch 'David Lynch Explains TM' on YouTube YES ☐ NO ☐

3. Consider one last pre-marathon weekend blowout YES ☐ NO ☐

As I prepare to close my eyes at the
end of WEEK 8, I am grateful for:

1 ....

2 ....

3 ....

Next week in my training I aim to be
1 PER CENT better at:

....

pen/pencil down, lights out, 3 deep breaths

WEEK 8 OFFICIALLY SMASHED

tick box

Week 9

HALFWAY FEELS GOOD!

AT A GLANCE:

Tues: 40 mins EASY RUN

Thurs: 48 mins JOG/TEMPO RUN/
EASY RUN/WALK

Sat: 60 mins WALK/RUN

Sun: 120 mins WALK/JOG

TOTAL TRAINING TIME: 4 hrs 28 mins

(TWO MINUTES LESS THAN LAST WEEK!!)

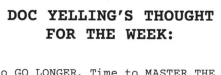

DOC YELLING'S THOUGHT FOR THE WEEK:

Time to GO LONGER. Time to MASTER THE MILES.
Wow, look at you!!! Welcome to phase 3, the most
important four weeks of your entire marathon schedule.
You now KNOW you can run longer. Long runs are where
you now live. Make sure you really listen to your body
from here on in. Break it and you'll never make it.
What is it telling you with regards to working
out your optimal marathon pace?

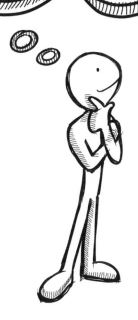

DAY
57

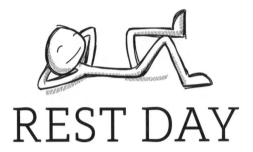

REST DAY

DON'T

THINK

ABOUT RUNNING

OR

ANYTHING

TO

DO

WITH

RUNNING

AT

ALL

(SEE YOU TOMORROW)

DAY 57: **COOL!** ☐

tick box

Week 9: Monday: _ _ /_ _ /_ _

Woke up at: _ _ /_ _ am/pm
In bed now: _ _ /_ _ am/pm

Today I ate: OK ☐ WELL ☐ AWESOME ☐
My water intake was: OK ☐ GOOD ☐ AWESOME ☐
As a human I was: KIND ☐ THOUGHTFUL ☐ PRESENT ☐

Tomorrow I aim to be 1% better at:

: ....
: ....
: ....

As I prepare to close my eyes
I am grateful for:

: ....
: ....
: ....

pen/pencil down
lights out
3 deep breaths

Only **62** days to go ➡ ➡ ➡

DAY
58

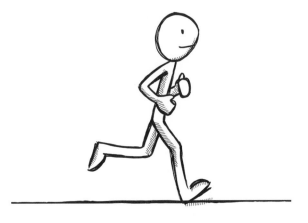

40 mins easy run

NOTES:

Location: ....

Weather: ....

Time start: _ _ /_ _ am/pm

Time finish: _ _ /_ _ am/pm

DAY 58: **SUPER COOL!**

tick box

Week 9: Tuesday: _ _ /_ _ /_ _

Woke up at: _ _ /_ _ am/pm
In bed now: _ _ /_ _ am/pm

Today I ate: OK ☐ WELL ☐ AWESOME ☐
My water intake was: OK ☐ GOOD ☐ AWESOME ☐
As a human I was: KIND ☐ THOUGHTFUL ☐ PRESENT ☐

Tomorrow I aim to be 1% better at:

: ....
: ....
: ....

As I prepare to close my eyes
I am grateful for:

: ....
: ....
: ....

pen/pencil down
lights out
3 deep breaths

Only **61** days to go ➡➡➡

Rest Day/X-Train Day

A fun thing to do this week is experiment with an alternative 'go-to' walk/run. Even something that might feel a bit silly at first.

This can be helpful on ever longer runs to give your body a break from the same repetitive movement. I have found shaking things up a bit for, say, 5 to 10 minutes every hour or so when I'm going L-O-N-G, to be highly effective in fending off stiffness, cramp and general all-round maranoia.

My adopted method of taking half a mile off (which I now do every fifth/sixth mile during a long run/race, regardless) is something I refer to as the South Bank Scuttle.

This is named in honour of a petite lady I saw one day when I was on the way to work. She appeared to be mesmerically gliding along the South Bank of the River Thames, with exceedingly high cadence but minimal arm and leg movement combined with barely any foot lift.

As she passed me FOR THE THIRD TIME, her technique looked so effortless and efficient, I simply had to have a go. The South Bank Scuttle is now officially my 'go-to' failsafe when I want to take a break from running but not lose any time.

EUREKA!!

DAY 59: **THE COOLEST!**

tick box

Week 9: Wednesday: _ _ /_ _ /_ _

Woke up at: _ _ /_ _ am/pm
In bed now: _ _ /_ _ am/pm

Today I ate: **OK** ☐ WELL ☐ AWESOME ☐
My water intake was: **OK** ☐ GOOD ☐ AWESOME ☐
As a human I was: KIND ☐ THOUGHTFUL ☐ PRESENT ☐

Tomorrow I aim to be 1% better at:

: ....

: ....

: ....

As I prepare to close my eyes
I am grateful for:

: ....

: ....

: ....

pen/pencil down
lights out
3 deep breaths

Only **60** days to go ➡ ➡ ➡ ➡

DAY
60

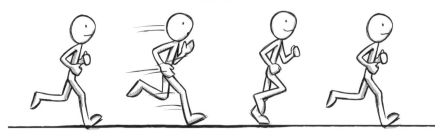

10 mins easy run/
(4 mins tempo run,
3 mins easy jog/walk recovery)
x 4/10 mins easy run
= 48 mins total

NOTES:

Location: ....
Weather: ....
Time start: _ _ /_ _ am/pm
Time finish: _ _ /_ _ am/pm

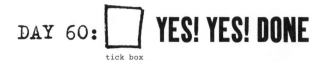

DAY 60: YES! YES! DONE

tick box

Week 9: Thursday: _ _ /_ _ /_ _

Woke up at: _ _ /_ _ am/pm
In bed now: _ _ /_ _ am/pm

Today I ate: OK ☐ WELL ☐ AWESOME ☐
My water intake was: OK ☐ GOOD ☐ AWESOME ☐
As a human I was: KIND ☐ THOUGHTFUL ☐ PRESENT ☐

Tomorrow I aim to be 1% better at:

: ....
: ....
: ....

As I prepare to close my eyes
I am grateful for:

: ....
: ....
: ....

pen/pencil down
lights out
3 deep breaths

Only **59** days to go ➡➡➡➡

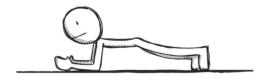

Rest Day/X-Train Day

KINDNESS FRIDAY THOUGHT:

DEAR BRAIN,

Have we had any more thoughts about meditation?

What are we frightened of?

What do we have to lose?

Why don't we check out Evans's top 3 meditation YouTube go-tos?

1. Sitting Together in Presence:
A Meditation with Eckhart Tolle

2. 5-Minute Meditation Anyone Can Do Anywhere:
Re-centre & Clear Your Mind with Boho Beautiful

3. Beautiful Guided Meditation with Mooji:
A Peaceful Life Is Priceless

DAY 61: TiCK-TOCK YAH!

tick box

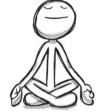

Week 9: Friday: _ _ /_ _ /_ _

Woke up at: _ _ /_ _ am/pm
In bed now: _ _ /_ _ am/pm

Today I ate: OK ☐ WELL ☐ AWESOME ☐
My water intake was: OK ☐ GOOD ☐ AWESOME ☐
As a human I was: KIND ☐ THOUGHTFUL ☐ PRESENT ☐

Tomorrow I aim to be 1% better at:

: ....
: ....
: ....

As I prepare to close my eyes
I am grateful for:

: ....
: ....
: ....

pen/pencil down
lights out
3 deep breaths

Only **58** days to go ➡ ➡ ➡ ➡

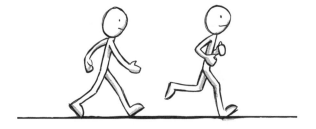

60 mins walk/run

Watch (and join in with) this video on YouTube before you go for a run today:

GUIDED WIM HOF METHOD BREATHING

Then before you move (but after you have finished!), take a good minute (or even two!) to give thanks once again for the cause for which you are running. To be given the chance to be able to do something for someone else while at the same time improving who you are forever is one of the greatest blessings a person can have come their way.

'If your WHY is big enough, you'll always find a HOW.'

Said someone very wise somewhere, once.

NOW, get out there and enjoy your BEST Saturday training session EVER!

Location: ....

Weather: ....

Time start: _ _ /_ _ am/pm

Time finish: _ _ /_ _ am/pm

DAY 62:

☐
tick box

NAiLED!

Week 9: Saturday: _ _ /_ _ /_ _

Woke up at: _ _ /_ _ am/pm
In bed now: _ _ /_ _ am/pm

Today I ate: OK ☐ WELL ☐ AWESOME ☐

My water intake was: OK ☐ GOOD ☐ AWESOME ☐

As a human I was: KIND ☐ THOUGHTFUL ☐ PRESENT ☐

Tomorrow I aim to be 1% better at:

: ....
: ....
: ....

As I prepare to close my eyes
I am grateful for:

: ....
: ....
: ....

pen/pencil down
lights out
3 deep breaths

Only **57** days to go ➡➡➡

LONG **DAY 63** RUN

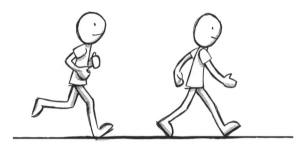

(28 mins run, 2 mins walk) x 4
= 2 hrs total
Or distance goal: 10 to 12 miles

YOUR NINTH LONG-RUN DAY!

LONG RUN NUMBER 9

Location: ....

Weather: ....

Time start: _ _ /_ _ am/pm

Time finish: _ _ /_ _ am/pm

Mood before: ....

Mood after: ....

WRITE DOWN FIVE WORDS TO DESCRIBE YOUR DAY TODAY:

1. ....
2. ....
3. ....

4. ....
5. ....

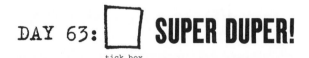

DAY 63: ☐ **SUPER DUPER!**

tick box

Week 9: Sunday: _ _ /_ _ /_ _

NIGHTY NIGHT WEEK 9

Woke up at: _ _ /_ _ am/pm
In bed now: _ _ /_ _ am/pm

This week my diet has been OK ☐ PRETTY GOOD ☐ AWESOME ☐

This week I have slept OK ☐ WELL ☐ AMAZINGLY ☐

This week my training has gone OK ☐ WELL ☐ AWESOMELY ☐

Going into WEEK 10 I will:

1. Experiment with an alternative 'go-to' walk/jog/run action YES ☐ NO ☐

2. Check in with my chosen charity and fund-raising efforts YES ☐ NO ☐

3. Research simple, useful breathing techniques YES ☐ NO ☐

As I prepare to close my eyes at the end of WEEK 9, I am grateful for:

1 ....

2 ....

3 ....

Next week in my training I aim to be 1 PER CENT better at:

....

pen/pencil down, lights out, 3 deep breaths

WEEK 9 OFFICiALLY SMASHED ☐

tick box

Week 10

GO GO GO!

AT A GLANCE:

Tues: 35 mins EASY RUN/
TEMPO RUN/RECOVERY

Thurs: 30 mins EASY RUN

Sat: EXTRA REST DAY!!

Sun: 2 hrs 30 mins to 3 hrs
HALF-MARATHON/LONG RUN

TOTAL TRAINING TIME:
3 hrs 35 mins to 4 hrs 5 mins

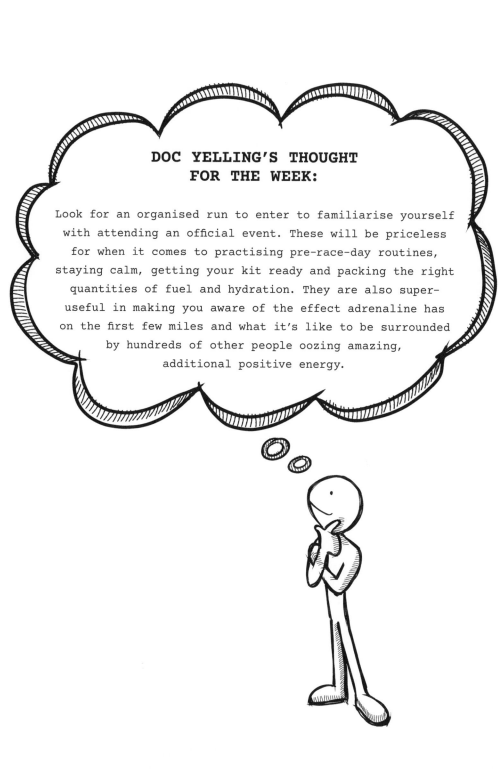

**DOC YELLING'S THOUGHT
FOR THE WEEK:**

Look for an organised run to enter to familiarise yourself
with attending an official event. These will be priceless
for when it comes to practising pre-race-day routines,
staying calm, getting your kit ready and packing the right
quantities of fuel and hydration. They are also super-
useful in making you aware of the effect adrenaline has
on the first few miles and what it's like to be surrounded
by hundreds of other people oozing amazing,
additional positive energy.

DAY
64

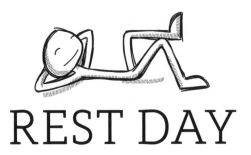

REST DAY

DON'T

THINK

ABOUT RUNNING

OR

ANYTHING

TO

DO

WITH

RUNNING

AT

ALL

(SEE YOU TOMORROW)

DAY 64: **RESTED!**

tick box

Week 10: Monday: _ _ /_ _ /_ _

Woke up at: _ _ /_ _ am/pm
In bed now: _ _ /_ _ am/pm

Today I ate: OK ☐ WELL ☐ AWESOME ☐
My water intake was: OK ☐ GOOD ☐ AWESOME ☐
As a human I was: KIND ☐ THOUGHTFUL ☐ PRESENT ☐

Tomorrow I aim to be 1% better at:

: ....
: ....
: ....

As I prepare to close my eyes
I am grateful for:

: ....
: ....
: ....

pen/pencil down
lights out
3 deep breaths

Only **55** days to go ➡➡➡

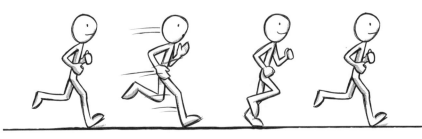

10 mins easy run/
3 x (3 mins tempo) with
3 x (2 mins jog recovery)/
10 mins easy run
= **35 mins total**

NOTES:

Location: ....

Weather: ....

Time start: _ _ /_ _ am/pm

Time finish: _ _ /_ _ am/pm

DAY 65: 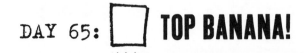 **TOP BANANA!**

tick box

Week 10: Tuesday: _ _ /_ _ /_ _

Woke up at: _ _ /_ _ am/pm
In bed now: _ _ /_ _ am/pm

Today I ate: OK ☐ WELL ☐ AWESOME ☐
My water intake was: OK ☐ GOOD ☐ AWESOME ☐
As a human I was: KIND ☐ THOUGHTFUL ☐ PRESENT ☐

Tomorrow I aim to be 1% better at:

: ....
: ....
: ....

As I prepare to close my eyes
I am grateful for:

: ....
: ....
: ....

pen/pencil down
lights out
3 deep breaths

Only **54** days to go ➡ ➡ ➡

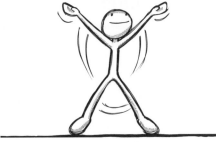

Rest Day/X-Train Day

POW! YOU'RE HEADING TOWARDS YOUR LONGEST RUN SO FAR.

THWACK! BRING ON THIS WEEKEND'S HALF-MARATHON.

KABOOM! PREPARE MAIN ENGINE START.

This is the week to begin immersing yourself in running lore. You are way past the halfway point in your training. Be the energy you want to feel on the start line in seven Sundays' time. Surround yourself between now and then with hacks, hints and inspiration from the best of the best.

Start by checking out my favourite YouTube running crew: www.therunexperience.com. They have multiple videos on breathing alone!

There are literally thousands of other fantastically helpful running gangs and gurus online. Many rabbit holes for you to get lost down! But do remember to come up for air now and again. I don't want to lose you along the way.

WHERE ATTENTION GOES, ENERGY GROWS!

DAY 66: **GADZOOKS!**

tick box

```
Week 10: Wednesday: _ _ /_ _ /_ _
```

Woke up at: _ _ /_ _ am/pm
In bed now: _ _ /_ _ am/pm

Today I ate: OK ☐ WELL ☐ AWESOME ☐
My water intake was: OK ☐ GOOD ☐ AWESOME ☐
As a human I was: KIND ☐ THOUGHTFUL ☐ PRESENT ☐

Tomorrow I aim to be 1% better at:

: ....
: ....
: ....

As I prepare to close my eyes
I am grateful for:

: ....
: ....
: ....

pen/pencil down
lights out
3 deep breaths

Only **53** days to go ➡ ➡ ➡ ➡

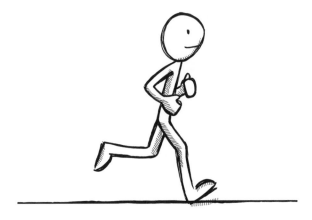

30 mins easy run

NOTES:

Location: ....

Weather: ....

Time start: _ _ /_ _ am/pm

Time finish: _ _ /_ _ am/pm

DAY 67: **HOT DOG!**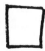

tick box

```
Week 10: Thursday: _ _ /_ _ /_ _
```

Woke up at: _ _ /_ _ am/pm
In bed now: _ _ /_ _ am/pm

Today I ate: **OK** ☐ WELL ☐ AWESOME ☐
My water intake was: **OK** ☐ GOOD ☐ AWESOME ☐
As a human I was: KIND ☐ THOUGHTFUL ☐ PRESENT ☐

Tomorrow I aim to be 1% better at:

: ....
: ....
: ....

As I prepare to close my eyes
I am grateful for:

: ....
: ....
: ....

pen/pencil down
lights out
3 deep breaths

Only **52** days to go ➡➡➡➡

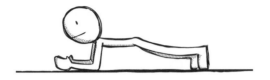

Rest Day/X-Train Day

FUN FRIDAY THOUGHT:

Long-run routes from now on.

As always, K.I.S.S. Keep it super simple. Once my long runs stretch over the 10-mile mark, I always keep to the exact same route (along the Thames Path and back), merely extending my weekend outings by a couple more miles week on week.

Out for six miles, back for six miles. Out for seven, back for seven.

I really like this method as, mentally, every mile counts double. If I'm two miles out, I have to get back somehow, regardless, therefore in my mind 1 mile counts for 2, 2 for 4, 4 for 8, and so on.

This weekend, once I'm over six and a half miles, all I have to do is turn round and before I know it I'll be home in no time, with a half-marathon under my belt. YOWZER!!

Personally, I prefer not to run with a watch for distance/pace and use landmarks instead, like bends in the river and various old, giant trees. If I want to know how long I've been out, I merely ask someone for the time. I'm old school, but hey, that's just me.

DAY 68: **PASSED!**

tick box

Week 10: Friday: _ _ /_ _ /_ _

Woke up at: _ _ /_ _ am/pm
In bed now: _ _ /_ _ am/pm

Today I ate: OK ☐ WELL ☐ AWESOME ☐
My water intake was: OK ☐ GOOD ☐ AWESOME ☐
As a human I was: KIND ☐ THOUGHTFUL ☐ PRESENT ☐

Tomorrow I aim to be 1% better at:

: ....
: ....
: ....

As I prepare to close my eyes
I am grateful for:

: ....
: ....
: ....

pen/pencil down
lights out
3 deep breaths

Only **51** days to go ➡ ➡ ➡ ➡

DAY
69

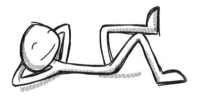

BONUS REST DAY

WHAT'S THIS??

A bonus rest day! How very dare the Great Doctor!! Is he getting soft in his old age or what??

Obviously, I'm joking. DOC YELLING IS THE KING OF THE TRAINING PLAN. If the Great Doctor says rest, WE REST, PEOPLE!!

TOP 10 INSPIRATIONAL MOVIES TO WATCH WHILE VEGGING OUT ON THE COUCH THE DAY BEFORE A BIG RUN

1. The Barkley Marathons
2. Breaking 2
3. Free Solo
4. Forrest Gump
5. Running on the Sun

6. The Dawn Wall
7. Chariots of Fire
8. 3100: Run and Become
9. Spirit of the Marathon
10. Boston: The Documentary

(I also really like Rise of the Sufferfests, but no one else seems to agree with me, so I left it out.)

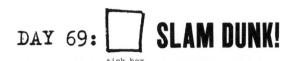

DAY 69: ☐ **SLAM DUNK!**

tick box

```
┌─────────────────────────────────────────┐
│  Week 10: Saturday: _ _ /_ _ /_ _        │
└─────────────────────────────────────────┘
```

Woke up at: _ _ /_ _ am/pm
In bed now: _ _ /_ _ am/pm

Today I ate: OK ☐ WELL ☐ AWESOME ☐
My water intake was: OK ☐ GOOD ☐ AWESOME ☐
As a human I was: KIND ☐ THOUGHTFUL ☐ PRESENT ☐

Tomorrow I aim to be 1% better at:

: ....
: ....
: ....

As I prepare to close my eyes
I am grateful for:

: ....
: ....
: ....

pen/pencil down
lights out
3 deep breaths

Only **50** days to go ➡➡➡

LONG **DAY 70** RUN

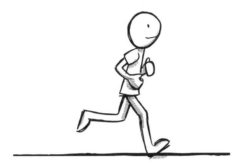

Race Half-Marathon
Or long run 2 hrs 30 mins
Or distance goal: 12 to 14 miles

YOUR TENTH LONG–RUN DAY!

LONG RUN NUMBER 10

Location: ....

Weather: ....

Time start: _ _ / _ _ am/pm

Time finish: _ _ / _ _ am/pm

Mood before: ....

Mood after: ....

WRITE DOWN FIVE WORDS TO DESCRIBE YOUR DAY TODAY:

1. ....
2. ....
3. ....

4. ....
5. ....

DAY 70: **BEAUTiFUL!**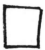

tick box

Week 10: Sunday: _ _ /_ _ /_ _

NIGHTY NIGHT WEEK 10

Woke up at: _ _ /_ _ am/pm
In bed now: _ _ /_ _ am/pm

This week my diet has been OK ☐ PRETTY GOOD ☐ AWESOME ☐

This week I have slept OK ☐ WELL ☐ AMAZINGLY ☐

This week my training has gone OK ☐ WELL ☐ AWESOMELY ☐

Going into WEEK 11 I will:

1. Begin watching short running/coaching/hack videos YES ☐ NO ☐

2. Start making a plan for my longer runs YES ☐ NO ☐

3. Give myself a massive pat on the back for my
   half-marathon YES ☐ NO ☐

As I prepare to close my eyes at the
end of WEEK 10, I am grateful for:

1 ....

2 ....

3 ....

Next week in my training I aim to be
1 PER CENT better at:

....

pen/pencil down, lights out, 3 deep breaths

WEEK 10 OFFiCiALLY SMASHED

tick box

Week 11

BRiNG iT ON!

AT A GLANCE:

Tues: 40 mins EASY RUN

Thurs: 50 mins EASY RUN

Sat: 60 mins EASY WALK/RUN

Sun: 2 hrs 30 mins to 3 hrs
HALF-MARATHON/
LONG RUN

TOTAL TRAINING TIME:
5 hrs to 5 hrs 30 mins

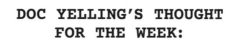

DOC YELLING'S THOUGHT
FOR THE WEEK:

Steady running only this week, please. Focus
on staying calm the whole time you're out there.
The running is the thing. Get lost in the process.
The miles happen automatically. Drop in a few miles
at what you think might be your marathon pace
whenever you feel comfortable. Keep your form: hips
high, chin level, shoulders square. Look upwards
and forwards. Onwards!

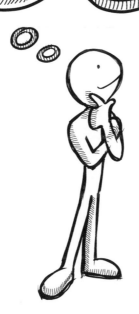

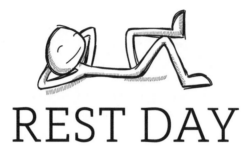

REST DAY

DON'T

THINK

ABOUT RUNNING

OR

ANYTHING

TO

DO

WITH

RUNNING

AT

ALL

(SEE YOU TOMORROW)

DAY 71: **CLASS!**

tick box

Week 11: Monday: _ _ /_ _ /_ _

Woke up at: _ _ /_ _ am/pm
In bed now: _ _ /_ _ am/pm

Today I ate: OK ☐ WELL ☐ AWESOME ☐
My water intake was: OK ☐ GOOD ☐ AWESOME ☐
As a human I was: KIND ☐ THOUGHTFUL ☐ PRESENT ☐

Tomorrow I aim to be 1% better at:

: ....
: ....
: ....

As I prepare to close my eyes
I am grateful for:

: ....
: ....
: ....

pen/pencil down
lights out
3 deep breaths

Only **48** days to go ➡ ➡ ➡ ➡

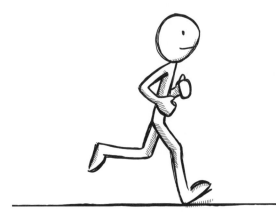

40 mins easy run

```
    Location: ........................
     Weather: ........................
  Time start: _ _ /_ _ am/pm
 Time finish: _ _ /_ _ am/pm
```

DAY 72: **BAGGED!**

tick box

```
Week 11: Tuesday: _ _ /_ _ /_ _
```

Woke up at: _ _ /_ _ am/pm
In bed now: _ _ /_ _ am/pm

Today I ate: OK ☐ WELL ☐ AWESOME ☐
My water intake was: OK ☐ GOOD ☐ AWESOME ☐
As a human I was: KIND ☐ THOUGHTFUL ☐ PRESENT ☐

Tomorrow I aim to be 1% better at:

: ....
: ....
: ....

As I prepare to close my eyes
I am grateful for:

: ....
: ....
: ....

pen/pencil down
lights out
3 deep breaths

Only **47** days to go ➡ ➡ ➡ ➡

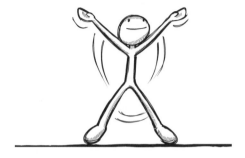

Rest Day/X-Train Day

DEAR BRAIN,

How was Sunday for us?

What did we learn?

`F.W.I.W.:` Where are we with hills and slopes? After my first few marathons/half-marathons, I realised that trying to run up anything even remotely resembling a slope (let alone an actual hill) was entirely counterproductive for someone of my ability. I found running/jogging, shuffling even, ten times more exhausting than merely walking/yomping up the slope, yet only fractionally quicker (if at all!!).

Hence, ever since this epiphany, I never run up slopes or hills at all anymore. At my race pace, it has no detrimental effect on my time whatsoever. In fact, on the contrary, if I walk up hills and then let my legs go on the way down, I can actually pick up the odd half-minute here and there!

WOO HOO - SOMEBODY STOP ME!!

DAY 73: TICK-TOCK, BABY!

tick box

Week 11: Wednesday: _ _ /_ _ /_ _

Woke up at: _ _ /_ _ am/pm
In bed now: _ _ /_ _ am/pm

Today I ate: OK ☐ WELL ☐ AWESOME ☐
My water intake was: OK ☐ GOOD ☐ AWESOME ☐
As a human I was: KIND ☐ THOUGHTFUL ☐ PRESENT ☐

Tomorrow I aim to be 1% better at:

: ....
: ....
: ....

As I prepare to close my eyes
I am grateful for:

: ....
: ....
: ....

pen/pencil down
lights out
3 deep breaths

Only **46** days to go ➡➡➡➡

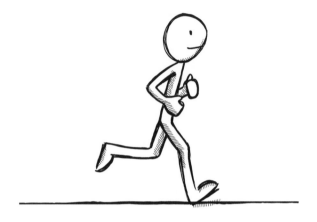

50 mins easy run

NOTES:

Location: ....
Weather: ....
Time start: _ _ /_ _ am/pm
Time finish: _ _ /_ _ am/pm

DAY 74: **CLOCKED!**

tick box

Woke up at: _ _ /_ _ am/pm
In bed now: _ _ /_ _ am/pm

Today I ate: OK ☐ WELL ☐ AWESOME ☐
My water intake was: OK ☐ GOOD ☐ AWESOME ☐
As a human I was: KIND ☐ THOUGHTFUL ☐ PRESENT ☐

Tomorrow I aim to be 1% better at:

: ....
: ....
: ....

As I prepare to close my eyes
I am grateful for:

: ....
: ....
: ....

pen/pencil down
lights out
3 deep breaths

Only **45** days to go ➡ ➡ ➡ ➡

DAY
75

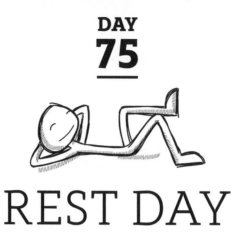

REST DAY

Tomorrow's 'easy' walk/run is 60 minutes, ahead of Sunday's long run. After this weekend, six more long runs and you will officially be a marathoner! YOUR SIXTH LONG RUN FROM NOW WILL BE YOUR ACTUAL MARATHON.

You've come so far, from here on in IT'S TIME TO PRIORITISE THE BASICS. As of this moment, 'EASY' really means E-A-S-Y. Don't even think about picking up the pace.

Use your remaining 'easy' sessions to shake down those gorgeous, lovely limbs of yours, listen to what they're telling you. Talk back to them. I do. Honestly. Out loud. Especially on a Saturday.

'EASY ... EASY ... EASY ...'

'Thank you, head. Thank you, neck. Thank you, shoulders. Thank you, arms. Thank you, hands. Thank you, stomach.'

'EASY ... EASY ... EASY ...'

'Thank you, bum. Thank you, thighs. Thank you, knees. Thank you, calves. Thank you, ankles. Thank you, feet. Thank you, toes.'

'EASY ... EASY ... EASY ...'

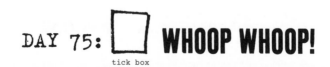

DAY 75: ☐ **WHOOP WHOOP!**

tick box

Woke up at: _ _ /_ _ am/pm
In bed now: _ _ /_ _ am/pm

Today I ate: OK ☐ WELL ☐ AWESOME ☐
My water intake was: OK ☐ GOOD ☐ AWESOME ☐
As a human I was: KIND ☐ THOUGHTFUL ☐ PRESENT ☐

Tomorrow I aim to be 1% better at:

: ....
: ....
: ....

As I prepare to close my eyes
I am grateful for:

: ....
: ....
: ....

pen/pencil down
lights out
3 deep breaths

Only **44** days to go ➡➡➡➡

DAY
76

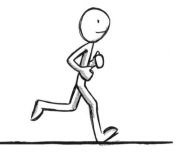

60 mins easy walk/run

EASY. EASY. EASY.

Thank you. Thank you. Thank you.

EASY. EASY. EASY.

Thank you. Thank you. Thank you.

EASY. EASY. EASY.

Thank you. Thank you. Thank you.

EASY. EASY. EASY.

```
Location: ..........................
Weather: ..........................
Time start: _ _ /_ _ am/pm
Time finish: _ _ /_ _ am/pm
```

DAY 76: PERFECT!

tick box

```
Week 11: Saturday: _ _ /_ _ /_ _
```

Woke up at: _ _ /_ _ am/pm
In bed now: _ _ /_ _ am/pm

Today I ate: **OK** ☐ WELL ☐ AWESOME ☐
My water intake was: **OK** ☐ GOOD ☐ AWESOME ☐
As a human I was: KIND ☐ THOUGHTFUL ☐ PRESENT ☐

Tomorrow I aim to be 1% better at:

: ....
: ....
: ....

As I prepare to close my eyes
I am grateful for:

: ....
: ....
: ....

pen/pencil down
lights out
3 deep breaths

Only **43** days to go ➡➡➡

LONG **DAY 77** RUN

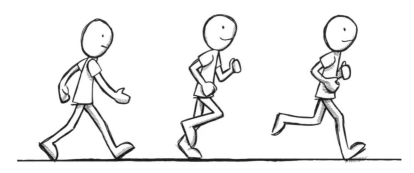

14 to 16 miles walk some/ jog some/run some

YOUR ELEVENTH LONG-RUN DAY!

LONG RUN NUMBER 11

Location: ....

Weather: ....

Time start: _ _ /_ _ am/pm

Time finish: _ _ /_ _ am/pm

Mood before: ....

Mood after: ....

WRITE DOWN FIVE WORDS TO DESCRIBE YOUR DAY TODAY:

1. ....
2. ....
3. ....

4. ....
5. ....

DAY 77: 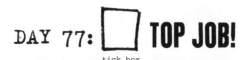 **TOP JOB!**

tick box

Week 11: Sunday: _ _ /_ _ /_ _

NIGHTY NIGHT WEEK 11

Woke up at: _ _ /_ _ am/pm

In bed now: _ _ /_ _ am/pm

This week my diet has been OK ☐ PRETTY GOOD ☐ AWESOME ☐

This week I have slept OK ☐ WELL ☐ AMAZINGLY ☐

This week my training has gone OK ☐ WELL ☐ AWESOMELY ☐

Going into WEEK 12 I will:

1. Focus on my uphill and downhill pacing YES ☐ NO ☐

2. Remember to prioritise the basics YES ☐ NO ☐

3. Decide to change my running shoes now or stick with the ones I have YES ☐ NO ☐

As I prepare to close my eyes at the end of WEEK 11, I am grateful for:

1 ....

2 ....

3 ....

Next week in my training I aim to be 1 PER CENT better at:

....

pen/pencil down, lights out, 3 deep breaths

WEEK 11 OFFICIALLY SMASHED

tick box

6
WEEKS
TO
GO

THE TEN COMMANDMENTS OF THE LAST SIX WEEKS OF YOUR COLOSSAL MARATHON TRAINING EFFORT

(IN NO PARTICULAR ORDER, LIKE MOSES)

1. Thou shalt have decided thine target time.
2. Thou shalt therefore have also decided thine miles per minute run rate.
3. Thou shalt have realised thou cannot out-train a bad diet.
4. Thou shalt seriously think about knocking the booze on the head completely for the next 42 days. (It's only 42 days!!)
5. Thou shalt check in with thine chosen charity.
6. Thou shalt protect thine sleep window like thine life depends on it.
7. Thou shalt practise thine 7-minute X-TRAINING sessions three times a week (AND LOVE THEM!).
8. Thou shalt, from now on, only run in thine race-day shoes.
9. Thou shalt complete all thine long-run training sessions without exception, wherever humanly possible, in their entirety, save for unavoidable circumstances to the contrary.
10. Thou shalt be super-careful not to: stub thine toe getting up for a pee in the middle of the night; turn thine ankle running for a bus or doing the garden (the weeds can wait); or acquiring any other similar, unnecessary, non-running-related injury that might jeopardise all the hard work thou hast put into thine titan marathon effort thus far.

Week 12

HELL YEAH!

AT A GLANCE:

Tues: 45 mins EASY RUN

Thurs: 60 mins EASY RUN/TEMPO RUN/ JOG/WALK

Sat: 60 mins RUN

Sun: 5 x (28 mins easy run + 2 mins walk) = 2 hrs 30 mins total

TOTAL TRAINING TIME: 5 to 6 hrs

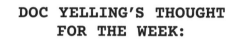

DOC YELLING'S THOUGHT
FOR THE WEEK:

Here come the proper long runs. The pressure may build
but it's all in the mind. Release the valve. To stay
disciplined is to stay calm. A realistic, achievable
pace and effort combination is vital. What feels like
an easy pace at the start of a long run will feel much
harder as the run goes on. Your target pace 'should'
feel easy for as long as possible. Eleven-minute
miles get you home in 4 hrs 48 mins.
Not too shabby!!!

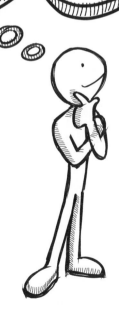

DAY
78

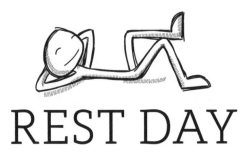

REST DAY

DON'T

THINK

ABOUT RUNNING

OR

ANYTHING

TO

DO

WITH

RUNNING

AT

ALL

(SEE YOU TOMORROW)

DAY 78: **AND RELAX!**

tick box

```
┌─────────────────────────────────────────┐
│                                         │
│   Week 12: Monday: _ _ /_ _ /_ _        │
│                                         │
└─────────────────────────────────────────┘
```

Woke up at: _ _ /_ _ am/pm
In bed now: _ _ /_ _ am/pm

Today I ate: OK ☐ WELL ☐ AWESOME ☐
My water intake was: OK ☐ GOOD ☐ AWESOME ☐
As a human I was: KIND ☐ THOUGHTFUL ☐ PRESENT ☐

Tomorrow I aim to be 1% better at:

: ....
: ....
: ....

As I prepare to close my eyes I am grateful for:

: ....
: ....
: ....

pen/pencil down
lights out
3 deep breaths

Only **41** days to go ➡➡➡➡

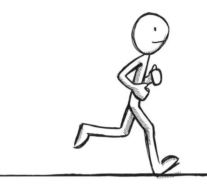

45 mins easy run

EASY ... EASY ... EASY ...

EASY ... EASY ... EASY ...

EASY ... EASY ... EASY ...

EASY ... EASY ... EASY ...

Location: ....

Weather: ....

Time start: _ _ /_ _ am/pm

Time finish: _ _ /_ _ am/pm

DAY 79: **BYE BYE, WE'RE DONE!**

tick box

Week 12: Tuesday: _ _ /_ _ /_ _

Woke up at: _ _ /_ _ am/pm
In bed now: _ _ /_ _ am/pm

Today I ate: OK ☐ WELL ☐ AWESOME ☐
My water intake was: OK ☐ GOOD ☐ AWESOME ☐
As a human I was: KIND ☐ THOUGHTFUL ☐ PRESENT ☐

Tomorrow I aim to be 1% better at:

: ....
: ....
: ....

As I prepare to close my eyes
I am grateful for:

: ....
: ....
: ....

pen/pencil down
lights out
3 deep breaths

Only **40** days to go ➡ ➡ ➡

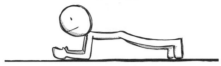

Rest day/
7-minute workout

TOP 5 MOST EXPENSIVE THINGS I OWN TO DO WITH RUNNING THAT WERE
DEFINITELY WORTH THE MONEY (I think):

1. My Apple iPod (£199)
2. My BEATS Powerbeats sports earphones (£129)
3. My Theragun Pro percussive massage device (£549)
4. My UK Saunas one-man infrared sauna (£989)
5. My NormaTec recovery boots (£1,195)

Note to reader: I have not been paid to mention/endorse any
of the above.

Note to manufacturers: I am happy to be paid to mention/endorse
any/all of the above.

Additional note to reader: If that ever happens, you'll be
the first to know.

Note to self: It's never going to happen. Ever.

(**Note to New Balance:** Thank you so much for my
running shoes, I adore them and swear by them.
They were, however, free and therefore could not
be included in the above 'paid for' list. That said,
I remain available to be considered as an official
'paid for' New Balance ambassador.)

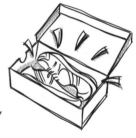

DAY 80: BOOM TiCK TiCK SHAKE THE ROOM!

tick box

Week 12: Wednesday: _ _ /_ _ /_ _

Woke up at: _ _ /_ _ am/pm
In bed now: _ _ /_ _ am/pm

Today I ate: OK ☐ WELL ☐ AWESOME ☐
My water intake was: OK ☐ GOOD ☐ AWESOME ☐
As a human I was: KIND ☐ THOUGHTFUL ☐ PRESENT ☐

Tomorrow I aim to be 1% better at:

: ....
: ....
: ....

As I prepare to close my eyes
I am grateful for:

: ....
: ....
: ....

pen/pencil down
lights out
3 deep breaths

Only **39** days to go ➡➡➡➡

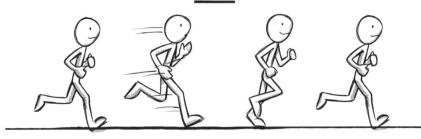

10 mins easy run/
40 mins (5 mins tempo run +
3 mins jog/walk recovery) x 5)/
10 mins easy run
= **60 mins total**

NOTES:

Location: ....

Weather: ....

Time start: _ _ /_ _ am/pm

Time finish: _ _ /_ _ am/pm

DAY 81: **SWEET!**

tick box

```
Week 12: Thursday: _ _ /_ _ /_ _
```

Woke up at: _ _ /_ _ am/pm
In bed now: _ _ /_ _ am/pm

Today I ate: OK ☐ WELL ☐ AWESOME ☐
My water intake was: OK ☐ GOOD ☐ AWESOME ☐
As a human I was: KIND ☐ THOUGHTFUL ☐ PRESENT ☐

Tomorrow I aim to be 1% better at:

: ....
: ....
: ....

As I prepare to close my eyes
I am grateful for:

: ....
: ....
: ....

pen/pencil down
lights out
3 deep breaths

Only **38** days to go ➡ ➡ ➡ ➡

Rest Day/X-Train Day

SUPER-HELPFUL, SUPER-WARM, SUPER-FUN
FRIDAY THOUGHT:

Create a 'go-to' gratitude roll of honour to help get you in the right mindset for each new mile come race day. I dedicated each mile of my first marathon to three little heroes I met soon after I started running.

'Jake. Sidney. Brandon. This next mile is for you. You are my heroes. You are my guys. Thank you. Thank you. Thank you.'

This year I'll be dedicating each new mile to members of the amazing team at Wexham Park Hospital, who looked after me after I was admitted to A&E in the middle of the night in February. I thought I had a trapped fart for most of the weekend until the pain became unbearable. Turned out I had a 6.5-mm kidney stone trying to sharp elbow its way down my ureter. Ouch. No, really, ouch.

Thank you: Shirley, Gaby, Dan, Sister Sue, Alex, Hazel, Violet, Rose, Fernando, Jessie, Louise, Juna, Molly, Mr Robinson, The great and powerful Mr Bhardwa, Paul from the RAF (who was helping out due to COVID). Plus, anyone else I may have met/talked to/annoyed but can't remember because I was pretty much out of it for the first few hours.

YOU ARE ALL AWESOME!!

DAY 82: SMASHED TO SMiTHEREENS!

tick box

```
Week 12: Friday: _ _ /_ _ /_ _
```

Woke up at: _ _ /_ _ am/pm
In bed now: _ _ /_ _ am/pm

Today I ate: OK ☐ WELL ☐ AWESOME ☐
My water intake was: OK ☐ GOOD ☐ AWESOME ☐
As a human I was: KIND ☐ THOUGHTFUL ☐ PRESENT ☐

Tomorrow I aim to be 1% better at:

: ....
: ....
: ....

**As I prepare to close my eyes
I am grateful for:**

: ....
: ....
: ....

pen/pencil down
lights out
3 deep breaths

Only **37** days to go ➡ ➡ ➡ ➡

DAY
83

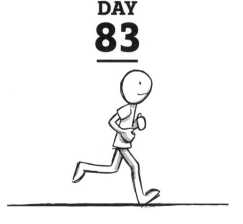

60 mins run/
target race pace

TRAIN HARD, FIGHT EASY
(SAS)

NOTES:

Location: ....
Weather: ....
Time start: _ _ /_ _ am/pm
Time finish: _ _ /_ _ am/pm

DAY 83: ☐ **KABLAMMO!**

tick box

```
Week 12: Saturday: _ _ /_ _ /_ _
```

Woke up at: _ _ /_ _ am/pm
In bed now: _ _ /_ _ am/pm

Today I ate: OK ☐ WELL ☐ AWESOME ☐
My water intake was: OK ☐ GOOD ☐ AWESOME ☐
As a human I was: KIND ☐ THOUGHTFUL ☐ PRESENT ☐

Tomorrow I aim to be 1% better at:

: ....
: ....
: ....

As I prepare to close my eyes
I am grateful for:

: ....
: ....
: ....

pen/pencil down
lights out
3 deep breaths

Only **36** days to go ➡ ➡ ➡

LONG **DAY 84** RUN

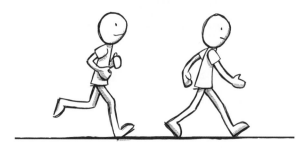

5 x (28 mins easy run + 2 mins walk)*
= 2 hrs 30 mins total
Or distance goal: 14 to 16 miles

*Include at least 8 miles at target marathon pace.

AND

Encourage yourself to take fewer (or even zero!) walking breaks
if you are feeling comfortable/strong/daring/experimental.

BE YOUR OWN GURU!

YOUR TWELFTH LONG-RUN DAY!

LONG RUN NUMBER 12

Location: ....

Weather: ....

Time start: _ _ /_ _ am/pm

Time finish: _ _ /_ _ am/pm

Mood before: ....

Mood after: ....

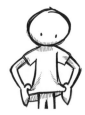

WHY NOT WEAR
YOUR OFFICIAL
RACE-DAY TOP
TO GET YOU IN
THE MOOD?

DAY 84: ☐ Hi-YAH! DONE!

tick box

Week 12: Sunday: _ _ /_ _ /_ _

NIGHTY NIGHT WEEK 12

Woke up at: _ _ /_ _ am/pm
In bed now: _ _ /_ _ am/pm

This week my diet has been OK ☐ PRETTY GOOD ☐ AWESOME ☐

This week I have slept OK ☐ WELL ☐ AMAZINGLY ☐

This week my training has gone OK ☐ WELL ☐ AWESOMELY ☐

Going into WEEK 13 I will:

1. Re-read the marathon runner's 10 Commandments YES ☐ NO ☐

2. Create my running angels' gratitude roll of honour YES ☐ NO ☐

3. Write to New Balance and tell them to make Evans an ambassador YES ☐ NO ☐

As I prepare to close my eyes at the
end of WEEK 12, I am grateful for:

1 ....

2 ....

3 ....

Next week in my training I aim to be
1 PER CENT better at:

....

pen/pencil down, lights out, 3 deep breaths

WEEK 12 OFFiCiALLY SMASHED ☐

tick box

Week 13

RUN, FORREST, RUN!

AT A GLANCE:

Tues: 50 mins EASY RUN

Thurs: 52 mins EASY RUN/TEMPO RUN/ JOG/WALK

Sat: 60 mins STEADY RUN

Sun: 3 hrs RUN/WALK

TOTAL TRAINING TIME: 6 hrs

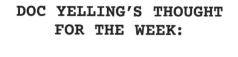

DOC YELLING'S THOUGHT
FOR THE WEEK:

Congratulations. No, seriously. You are now in deep. You have come a long way and thoroughly deserve to be here. The next two weeks are what this whole process is about. After that the taper kicks in and it's downhill all the way to the start line!!! Fourteen more days till then but only 8 training sessions, 2 more (seriously) long runs and then BOOM! Dig deep, this is it. But LISTEN TO YOUR BODY. Rest and recovery are key.

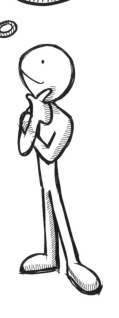

DAY
85

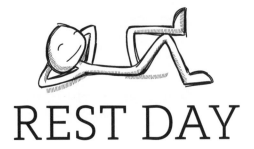

REST DAY

DON'T

THINK

ABOUT RUNNING

OR

ANYTHING

TO

DO

WITH

RUNNING

AT

ALL

(SEE YOU TOMORROW)

DAY 85: SEEN OFF!
tick box

Week 13: Monday: _ _ /_ _ /_ _

Woke up at: _ _ /_ _ am/pm
In bed now: _ _ /_ _ am/pm

Today I ate: OK ☐ WELL ☐ AWESOME ☐
My water intake was: OK ☐ GOOD ☐ AWESOME ☐
As a human I was: KIND ☐ THOUGHTFUL ☐ PRESENT ☐

Tomorrow I aim to be 1% better at:

: ....
: ....
: ....

As I prepare to close my eyes
I am grateful for:

: ....
: ....
: ....

pen/pencil down
lights out
3 deep breaths

Only **34** days to go ➡➡➡➡

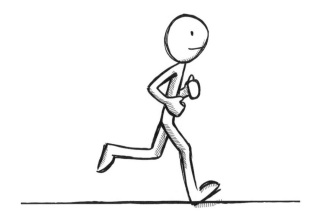

50 mins easy run

NOTES:

Location: ....
Weather: ....
Time start: _ _ /_ _ am/pm
Time finish: _ _ /_ _ am/pm

DAY 86: **CRACKiNG!**

tick box

Week 13: Tuesday: _ _ /_ _ /_ _

Woke up at: _ _ /_ _ am/pm
In bed now: _ _ /_ _ am/pm

Today I ate: OK ☐ WELL ☐ AWESOME ☐
My water intake was: OK ☐ GOOD ☐ AWESOME ☐
As a human I was: KIND ☐ THOUGHTFUL ☐ PRESENT ☐

Tomorrow I aim to be 1% better at:

: ....
: ....
: ....

As I prepare to close my eyes
I am grateful for:

: ....
: ....
: ....

pen/pencil down
lights out
3 deep breaths

Only **33** days to go ➡➡➡➡

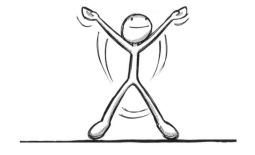

Rest Day/X-Train Day

A simple meditation from Brother Chris:

The closest I've ever come to what I imagine it might feel like to
be a monk is when I'm out running. The longer I'm out there, the
more monkish I feel.

I think it's because running (especially long-distance running)
really finds you out. The real YOU has no choice but to show up
sooner or later. Run for long enough and you will come face to
face with who you really are. How cool is that?

Perhaps this is also why long-distance runners have so much
respect for each other. We all know what a huge effort it takes
to make it to the start line, regardless of what our respective
times might be when we cross the finish line.

I find this profoundly moving, even just writing about it now.
I love being part of the running world. I hope you feel the same
way too.

GIVE YOURSELF A TICK JUST FOR THAT TODAY!

DAY 87: **DONE!** **OHMMMMM...**

tick box

```
Week 13: Wednesday: _ _ /_ _ /_ _
```

Woke up at: _ _ /_ _ am/pm
In bed now: _ _ /_ _ am/pm

Today I ate: OK ☐ WELL ☐ AWESOME ☐
My water intake was: OK ☐ GOOD ☐ AWESOME ☐
As a human I was: KIND ☐ THOUGHTFUL ☐ PRESENT ☐

Tomorrow I aim to be 1% better at:

: ....
: ....
: ....

As I prepare to close my eyes
I am grateful for:

: ....
: ....
: ....

pen/pencil down
lights out
3 deep breaths

Only **32** days to go ➡➡➡➡

DAY
88

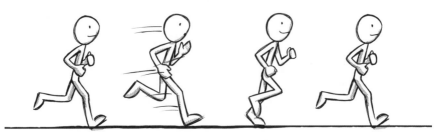

10 mins easy run/
32 mins of 4 x (6 mins tempo run,
2 mins easy jog/walk recovery)/
10 mins easy run
= 52 mins total

NOTES:

Location: ....
Weather: ....
Time start: _ _ /_ _ am/pm
Time finish: _ _ /_ _ am/pm

DAY 88:
tick box
BOOM SHAK A TiCK BOOM!

```
Week 13: Thursday: _ _ /_ _ /_ _
```

Woke up at: _ _ /_ _ am/pm
In bed now: _ _ /_ _ am/pm

Today I ate: OK ☐ WELL ☐ AWESOME ☐
My water intake was: OK ☐ GOOD ☐ AWESOME ☐
As a human I was: KIND ☐ THOUGHTFUL ☐ PRESENT ☐

Tomorrow I aim to be 1% better at:

: ....
: ....
: ....

As I prepare to close my eyes
I am grateful for:

: ....
: ....
: ....

pen/pencil down
lights out
3 deep breaths

Only **31** days to go ➥ ➥ ➥ ➥

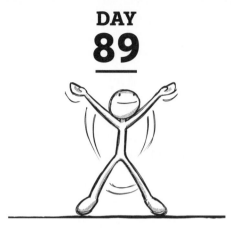

DAY
89

Rest Day/X-Train Day

I'm gonna stick with the monk theme this week, I kinda like it.

The sooner you unleash your inner monk on race day, the more pleasurable your whole experience will be. You have four more long runs between now and then to make sure you have her/him on speed dial.

Marathon Monkthink:

RELINQUISH THE EGO
RELEASE THE SPIRIT
EMBRACE THE PROCESS
TRUST THE RITUAL
LIVE THE REGIME
STAY HUMBLE YET CONFIDENT
STRONG YET RELAXED
FOCUSED YET OPEN-MINDED
SMILE THROUGH THE PAIN
CRY WITH JOY

BRING ON THE WEEKEND
AND DON'T FORGET TO BRING YOUR MONK!

DAY 89: ACHiEVED!

tick box

Week 13: Friday: _ _ /_ _ /_ _

Woke up at: _ _ /_ _ am/pm
In bed now: _ _ /_ _ am/pm

Today I ate: OK ☐ WELL ☐ AWESOME ☐
My water intake was: OK ☐ GOOD ☐ AWESOME ☐
As a human I was: KIND ☐ THOUGHTFUL ☐ PRESENT ☐

Tomorrow I aim to be 1% better at:

: ....
: ....
: ....

As I prepare to close my eyes
I am grateful for:

: ....
: ....
: ....

pen/pencil down
lights out
3 deep breaths

Only **30** days to go ➡➡➡➡

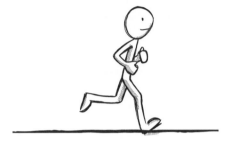

60 mins steady continuous run

MONK WEEK: THE FINALE

MY TOP 3 FAVOURITE YOUTUBE ACTUAL REAL MONKS:

1. Master Niels: First 3 Breathing Techniques
2. Yongey Mingyur Rinpoche: The Happiest Man on Earth
3. Master Shi Heng Yi: The 5 Hindrances to Self-Mastery

Watch Master Shi's 5 Hindrances TED TALK ahead of your long run tomorrow and tell me it didn't help! He's one badass of a Zen master.

NOTES:

Location: ....

Weather: ....

Time start: _ _ /_ _ am/pm

Time finish: _ _ /_ _ am/pm

DAY 90:

tick box

MONKED!

Week 13: Saturday: _ _ /_ _ /_ _

Woke up at: _ _ /_ _ am/pm
In bed now: _ _ /_ _ am/pm

Today I ate: OK ☐ WELL ☐ AWESOME ☐
My water intake was: OK ☐ GOOD ☐ AWESOME ☐
As a human I was: KIND ☐ THOUGHTFUL ☐ PRESENT ☐

Tomorrow I aim to be 1% better at:

: ....
: ....
: ....

As I prepare to close my eyes
I am grateful for:

: ....
: ....
: ....

pen/pencil down
lights out
3 deep breaths

Only **29** days to go ➡➡➡➡

LONG **DAY** **91** **RUN**

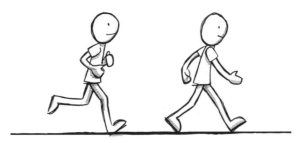

6 x (28 mins easy run, 2 mins walk)
= 3 hrs total
Or distance goal: 18 to 20 miles

Run continuously if you're confident to do so.
Include a few (6 to 8) miles at target marathon pace.

YOUR THIRTEENTH LONG-RUN DAY!

LONG RUN NUMBER 13

Location: ....

Weather: ....

Time start: _ _ /_ _ am/pm

Time finish: _ _ /_ _ am/pm

Mood before: ....

Mood after: ....

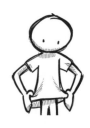

REMEMBER
TO WEAR
YOUR OFFICIAL
RACE-DAY TOP!

WRITE DOWN FIVE WORDS TO DESCRIBE YOUR DAY TODAY:

1. ....
2. ....
3. ....

4. ....
5. ....

DAY 91: **SEE YA! BOOM!**

tick box

Week 13: Sunday: _ _ /_ _ /_ _

NIGHTY NIGHT WEEK 13

Woke up at: _ _ /_ _ am/pm
In bed now: _ _ /_ _ am/pm

This week my diet has been OK ☐ PRETTY GOOD ☐ AWESOME ☐

This week I have slept OK ☐ WELL ☐ AMAZINGLY ☐

This week my training has gone OK ☐ WELL ☐ AWESOMELY ☐

Going into WEEK 14 I will:

1. Release my inner monk YES ☐ NO ☐

2. Release my inner monk YES ☐ NO ☐

3. Release my inner monk YES ☐ NO ☐

As I prepare to close my eyes at the
end of WEEK 13, I am grateful for:

1 ....

2 ....

3 ....

Next week in my training I aim to be
1 PER CENT better at:

....

pen/pencil down, lights out, 3 deep breaths

WEEK 13 OFFiCiALLY SMASHED ☐

tick box

Week 14

LEG's GO!

AT A GLANCE:

Tues: 50 mins EASY RUN

Thurs: 50 mins EASY RUN/STEADY/
RACE-PACE/TEMPO RUN/EASY RUN

Sat: 60 mins EASY WALK/RUN

Sun: 3 to 4 hrs LONG RUN

TOTAL TRAINING TIME: 6 to 7 hrs

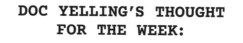

DOC YELLING'S THOUGHT
FOR THE WEEK:

When you truly believe you can do something, your
chances of achieving whatever that is rocket
exponentially. Now you KNOW you can smash a long run,
imagine the supercharging effect that's having on your
psyche. Two more long runs, the taper and then it's
race day. Focus, plan, prepare. Start off long runs
a minute off target pace, ease into it from
there, keep it up for 5 to 10 miles and
then ease off again.

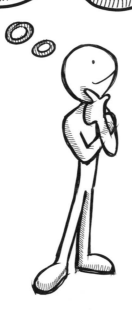

DAY
92

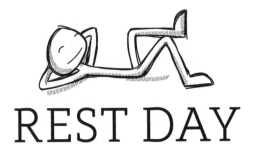

REST DAY

DON'T

THINK

ABOUT RUNNING

OR

ANYTHING

TO

DO

WITH

RUNNING

AT

ALL

(SEE YOU TOMORROW)

DAY 92: TiCKED OFF!

tick box

```
Week 14: Monday: _ _ /_ _ /_ _
```

Woke up at: _ _ /_ _ am/pm
In bed now: _ _ /_ _ am/pm

Today I ate: OK ☐ WELL ☐ AWESOME ☐
My water intake was: OK ☐ GOOD ☐ AWESOME ☐
As a human I was: KIND ☐ THOUGHTFUL ☐ PRESENT ☐

Tomorrow I aim to be 1% better at:

: ....
: ....
: ....

As I prepare to close my eyes
I am grateful for:

: ....
: ....
: ....

pen/pencil down
lights out
3 deep breaths

Only **27** days to go ➡ ➡ ➡

DAY
93

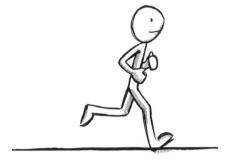

50 mins easy run

EASY ... EASY ... EASY ...

EASY ... EASY ... EASY ...

EASY ... EASY ... EASY ...

You know the routine by now. How good do these Tuesday morning easy runs feel? You continue to be AWESOME!!

NOTES:

Location: ....

Weather: ....

Time start: _ _ /_ _ am/pm

Time finish: _ _ /_ _ am/pm

DAY 93:

tick box

BOOOOOM!

Week 14: Tuesday: _ _ /_ _ /_ _

Woke up at: _ _ /_ _ am/pm
In bed now: _ _ /_ _ am/pm

Today I ate: OK ☐ WELL ☐ AWESOME ☐
My water intake was: OK ☐ GOOD ☐ AWESOME ☐
As a human I was: KIND ☐ THOUGHTFUL ☐ PRESENT ☐

Tomorrow I aim to be 1% better at:

: ....
: ....
: ....

As I prepare to close my eyes
I am grateful for:

: ....
: ....
: ....

pen/pencil down
lights out
3 deep breaths

Only **26** days to go ➡ ➡ ➡ ➡

DAY
94

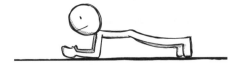

Rest Day/X-Train Day

DEAR BRAIN,

Thank you for all your help, support, patience and wisdom,
you've been amazing. Please help me remember:

CALM, PATIENCE,
CONFIDENCE, CALM
THE SUREFIRE WAY
TO DO NO HARM
WE'RE NEARLY THERE
WE'RE NEARLY DONE
WE'RE HEADING TOWARDS
OUR LAST LONG RUN

OUR LAST LONG RUN
BEFORE THE RACE
OUR FINAL CHANCE
TO FEEL THE PACE
THE PACE THAT'S RIGHT
THAT'S RIGHT FOR US
THE PACE THAT SPARKS
THAT INNER BUZZ

OF CALM, PATIENCE
CONFIDENCE, CALM
THE SUREFIRE WAY
TO DO NO HARM

DAY 94: CALMED AND TICKED!

tick box

Week 14: Wednesday: _ _ /_ _ /_ _

Woke up at: _ _ /_ _ am/pm
In bed now: _ _ /_ _ am/pm

Today I ate: OK ☐ WELL ☐ AWESOME ☐
My water intake was: OK ☐ GOOD ☐ AWESOME ☐
As a human I was: KIND ☐ THOUGHTFUL ☐ PRESENT ☐

Tomorrow I aim to be 1% better at:

: ....
: ....
: ....

As I prepare to close my eyes
I am grateful for:

: ....
: ....
: ....

pen/pencil down
lights out
3 deep breaths

Only **25** days to go ➡➡➡➡

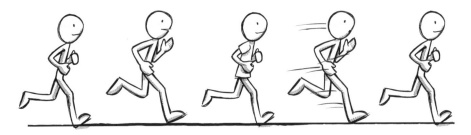

10 mins easy run/10 mins steady, 10 mins at race pace, 10 mins tempo run/10 mins easy run
= 50 mins total

THIS IS A TRULY FUN 50-MINUTE SESSION.

Look at that for a recipe (ALL HAIL THE GREAT DOC YELLING!!).
It's all in there. Everything you've ever wanted.
A microcosm of all the different disciplines you've built up,
brick by brick, over the last three months.

> NOTES:

Location: ....

Weather: ....

Time start: _ _ /_ _ am/pm

Time finish: _ _ /_ _ am/pm

DAY 95:

tick box

ABSOLUTELY LOVED iT!

```
Week 14: Thursday: _ _ /_ _ /_ _
```

Woke up at: _ _ /_ _ am/pm
In bed now: _ _ /_ _ am/pm

Today I ate: OK ☐ WELL ☐ AWESOME ☐
My water intake was: OK ☐ GOOD ☐ AWESOME ☐
As a human I was: KIND ☐ THOUGHTFUL ☐ PRESENT ☐

Tomorrow I aim to be 1% better at:

: ....
: ....
: ....

As I prepare to close my eyes
I am grateful for:

: ....
: ....
: ....

pen/pencil down
lights out
3 deep breaths

Only **24** days to go ➡➡➡➡

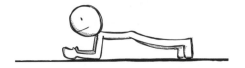

Rest Day/X-Train Day

PROFOUND FUNKY FUN FRIDAY THOUGHT:

This is your fourth-last weekend to race day. This is your last (really) long run before race day. This may be THE LAST TIME YOU EVER DO THIS. You may NEVER have a last (really) long-run training weekend again EVER in your life.

That is a MASSIVELY inspirational and important thought to meditate on. And here comes another ...

EVERYTHING you do between now and race day, you may NEVER do again. So MAKE THE ABSOLUTE MOST OF EVERY SECOND from now until the start line in 23 days' time.

Having made it this far, you have already proven you have what it takes to run a marathon. You may find that hard to believe, but I promise you it's true. From the moment you took that auspicious first step in training back in week one, you began filling up your running tanks with your own precious, priceless brand of running rocket fuel.

That's how this process works: you don't know you're doing it, until it's done. That's why Doc Yelling is a genius.

And so here we are. And here we go. One last long run. Just for show!

DAY 96: 5-4-3-2-1 WE HAVE LiFT OFF!

tick box

```
Week 14: Friday: _ _ /_ _ /_ _
```

Woke up at: _ _ /_ _ am/pm
In bed now: _ _ /_ _ am/pm

Today I ate: OK ☐ WELL ☐ AWESOME ☐
My water intake was: OK ☐ GOOD ☐ AWESOME ☐
As a human I was: KIND ☐ THOUGHTFUL ☐ PRESENT ☐

Tomorrow I aim to be 1% better at:

: ....
: ....
: ....

As I prepare to close my eyes
I am grateful for:

: ....
: ....
: ....

pen/pencil down
lights out
3 deep breaths

Only **23** days to go ➡ ➡ ➡ ➡

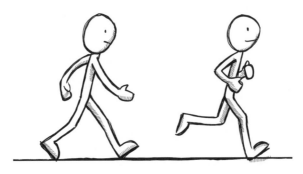

60 mins easy walk/run

BEST-EVER SATURDAY RUN THOUGHT:

REMEMBER: Even though you have one more big run tomorrow, the bulk of your training gold is already safely deposited in the Bank of Pheidippides! YOU'RE SO NEARLY DONE!! After tomorrow, it's literally downhill all the way to race day. Whoopee!

(Pheidippides is the reason we're all doing this. In case you didn't know, he's the Greek bloke who back in 490 BC ran from Marathon to Athens, 26 miles (ish), to announce to his fellow Athenians that the pesky invading Persians had been defeated. He then promptly collapsed and died. Poor chap.)

Location: ....

Weather: ....

Time start: _ _ /_ _ am/pm

Time finish: _ _ /_ _ am/pm

DAY 97:

tick box

MONSTERED!

```
Week 14: Saturday: _ _ /_ _ /_ _
```

Woke up at: _ _ /_ _ am/pm
In bed now: _ _ /_ _ am/pm

Today I ate: OK ☐ WELL ☐ AWESOME ☐
My water intake was: OK ☐ GOOD ☐ AWESOME ☐
As a human I was: KIND ☐ THOUGHTFUL ☐ PRESENT ☐

Tomorrow I aim to be 1% better at:

: ....
: ....
: ....

As I prepare to close my eyes
I am grateful for:

: ....
: ....
: ....

pen/pencil down
lights out
3 deep breaths

Only **22** days to go ➡➡➡

LONG **DAY 98** RUN

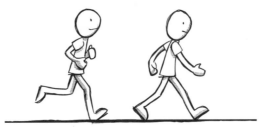

Longest distance run:
(28 mins easy, 2 mins walk) x 7
= 3 to 4 hrs total

DOC YELLING SAYS: Remember, people run at different paces so distance covered may be different. Run continuously if you're confident to do so. Or distance goal 20 to 22 miles.

YOUR FOURTEENTH LONG-RUN DAY!

LONG RUN NUMBER 14

Location: ....

Weather: ....

Time start: _ _ /_ _ am/pm

Time finish: _ _ /_ _ am/pm

Mood before: ....

Mood after: ....

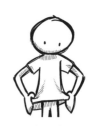

REMEMBER
TO WEAR
YOUR OFFICIAL
RACE-DAY TOP!

WRITE DOWN FIVE WORDS TO DESCRIBE YOUR DAY TODAY:

1. ....
2. ....
3. ....

4. ....
5. ....

DAY 98: YES PLEASE!

tick box

Week 14: Sunday: _ _ /_ _ /_ _

NIGHTY NIGHT WEEK 14

Woke up at: _ _ /_ _ am/pm
In bed now: _ _ /_ _ am/pm

This week my diet has been OK ☐ PRETTY GOOD ☐ AWESOME ☐

This week I have slept OK ☐ WELL ☐ AMAZINGLY ☐

This week my training has gone OK ☐ WELL ☐ AWESOMELY ☐

Going into WEEK 15 I will:

1. Reflect on all my training thus far, especially my final long run before race day YES ☐ NO ☐

2. Thank my brain for sticking up for me YES ☐ NO ☐

3. Thank my body for not falling apart YES ☐ NO ☐

As I prepare to close my eyes at the end of WEEK 14, I am grateful for:

1 ....

2 ....

3 ....

Next week in my training I aim to be 1 PER CENT better at:

....

pen/pencil down, lights out, 3 deep breaths

WEEK 14 OFFICIALLY SMASHED

tick box

Week 15

THE TAPER, WE LOVE THE TAPER!

AT A GLANCE:

Tues: 40 mins EASY RUN

Thurs: 50 mins EASY RUN/RACE PACE/ FASTER THAN RACE PACE

Sat: SECRET??

Sun: 2 hrs 10 mins EASY WALK/RUN

TOTAL TRAINING TIME: 3 hrs 40 mins

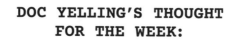

DOC YELLING'S THOUGHT
FOR THE WEEK:

Welcome to the taper. Where you 'need' to run
less to feel fresher, reach peak and get race ready.
DO NOT be tempted to throw in extra panic miles. At this
point they will have zero effect, put you at risk of being
tired on the start line and may even jeopardise your race
entirely. Get smart. Trust the training. Run your race
as often as you like in your mind (a good thing),
just not out on the road (a bad thing).

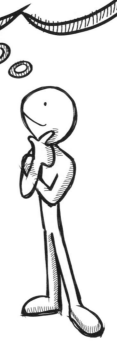

DAY
99

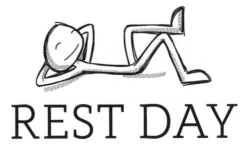

REST DAY

DON'T

THINK

ABOUT RUNNING

OR

ANYTHING

TO

DO

WITH

RUNNING

AT

ALL

(SEE YOU TOMORROW)

DAY 99: CHiLLED!

tick box

```
Week 15: Monday: _ _ /_ _ /_ _
```

Woke up at: _ _ /_ _ am/pm
In bed now: _ _ /_ _ am/pm

Today I ate: OK ☐ WELL ☐ AWESOME ☐
My water intake was: OK ☐ GOOD ☐ AWESOME ☐
As a human I was: KIND ☐ THOUGHTFUL ☐ PRESENT ☐

Tomorrow I aim to be 1% better at:

: ....
: ....
: ....

As I prepare to close my eyes
I am grateful for:

: ....
: ....
: ....

pen/pencil down
lights out
3 deep breaths

Only **20** days to go ➨➨➨➨

DAY
100

BOOM! BOOM! BOOM!

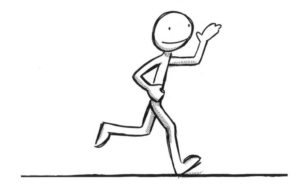

40 mins easy run

EASY ... 100 ... EASY ...

EASY ... 100 ... EASY ...

EASY ... 100 ... EASY ...

Location: ....

Weather: ....

Time start: _ _ /_ _ am/pm

Time finish: _ _ /_ _ am/pm

DAY 100: **CENTURY DONE BOOM!**

tick box

Woke up at: _ _ /_ _ am/pm
In bed now: _ _ /_ _ am/pm

Today I ate: OK ☐ WELL ☐ AWESOME ☐
My water intake was: OK ☐ GOOD ☐ AWESOME ☐
As a human I was: KIND ☐ THOUGHTFUL ☐ PRESENT ☐

Tomorrow I aim to be 1% better at:

: ....
: ....
: ....

As I prepare to close my eyes
I am grateful for:

: ....
: ....
: ....

pen/pencil down
lights out
3 deep breaths

Only **19** days to go ➡ ➡ ➡ ➡

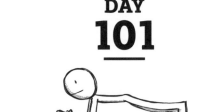

Rest Day/X-Train Day

THE REALLY HARD, PHYSICAL WORK IS ALL BUT DONE.
NOW IT'S TIME TO TURN DOWN THE NOISE.

Shhhhhhh.

For these last two and a bit weeks, really ENJOY dialling in your
pre-race-day prep.

Front load the non-running bases in your favour. You've met your
inner monk, now unleash your inner Zen master. Remember THE TITAN OF
PROCESS SLAYS THE PAUPER OF INTENTION. From now until race day give
religious attention to your marathon mindset and physical environment.
It will pay back a thousandfold in a couple of Sundays' time.

SUPER TIPS FROM THE JEDI MARATHON PLAYBOOK:

1. Begin to be a lot more conscious with regards to what and when
   you're eating/drinking.
2. Rest your legs whenever possible, wherever possible.
3. Keep the risk of needless injury somewhere between low and zero.
   The weeds, gardening AND ALL D.I.Y. can still wait!!
4. Only interact with people who love you, care for you, support
   you and want the best for you.
5. Watch/listen/read anything to do with amazing runners/people
   doing amazing running/peopley things whenever you have the time.

GO TO BED EARLIER THAN YOU HAVE DONE SINCE YOU WERE IN SCHOOL!!!

DAY 101: CHOP WOOD!/CARRY WATER!

tick box

Week 15: Wednesday: _ _ / _ _ / _ _

Woke up at: _ _ / _ _ am/pm
In bed now: _ _ / _ _ am/pm

Today I ate: **OK** ☐ WELL ☐ AWESOME ☐
My water intake was: **OK** ☐ GOOD ☐ AWESOME ☐
As a human I was: KIND ☐ THOUGHTFUL ☐ PRESENT ☐

Tomorrow I aim to be 1% better at:

: ....
: ....
: ....

As I prepare to close my eyes
I am grateful for:

: ....
: ....
: ....

pen/pencil down
lights out
3 deep breaths

Only **18** days to go ➡ ➡ ➡ ➡

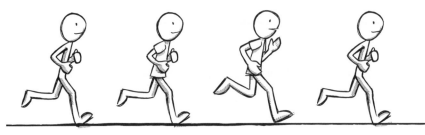

10 mins easy run/
30 mins run
(3 mins at marathon pace/
3 mins faster) x 5/
10 mins easy run
= 50 mins total

NOTES:

Location: ....

Weather: ....

Time start: _ _ /_ _ am/pm

Time finish: _ _ /_ _ am/pm

DAY 102: **SMASHED AND GRABBED!**

tick box

Week 15: Thursday: _ _ /_ _ /_ _

Woke up at: _ _ /_ _ am/pm
In bed now: _ _ /_ _ am/pm

Today I ate: OK ☐ WELL ☐ AWESOME ☐
My water intake was: OK ☐ GOOD ☐ AWESOME ☐
As a human I was: KIND ☐ THOUGHTFUL ☐ PRESENT ☐

Tomorrow I aim to be 1% better at:

: ....
: ....
: ....

As I prepare to close my eyes
I am grateful for:

: ....
: ....
: ....

pen/pencil down
lights out
3 deep breaths

Only **17** days to go ➡➡➡➡

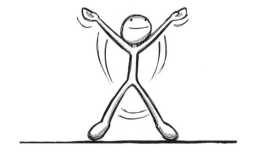

Rest Day/X-Train Day

OH MY GOD, I AM SO EXCITED FOR YOU!
MAYBE TOO EXCITED!!
YES, DEFINITELY TOO EXCITED!!

Which is really not what I should be advocating here, or anywhere
else for that matter. As I said on Wednesday, it really is time to
turn the noise down and keep it that way.

Shhhhhhh.

The thing is, I know what's around the corner and how much you're
going to love it. It's literally over the page.

GO ON, I DARE YOU, HAVE A LOOK.

IT'S ONLY AN EXTRA BLOOMIN'

Week 15: Friday: _ _ /_ _ /_ _

Woke up at: _ _ /_ _ am/pm
In bed now: _ _ /_ _ am/pm

Today I ate: OK ☐ WELL ☐ AWESOME ☐
My water intake was: OK ☐ GOOD ☐ AWESOME ☐
As a human I was: KIND ☐ THOUGHTFUL ☐ PRESENT ☐

Tomorrow I aim to be 1% better at:

: ....
: ....
: ....

As I prepare to close my eyes
I am grateful for:

: ....
: ....
: ....

pen/pencil down
lights out
3 deep breaths

Only **16** days to go ➡ ➡ ➡ ➡

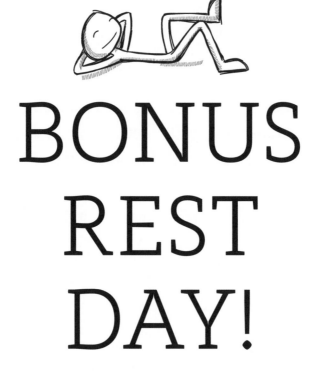

BONUS REST DAY!

FOLLOW DOC YELLING'S PRESCRIPTION INSTEAD:

1. Write down your race strategy and put it next to your bed.
2. Visualise, imagine and understand as much of your race plan as possible.
3. Be even MORE organised.
4. Use tomorrow's long run for any final race-pace tweaks.
5. Decide on your optimal kit, including gels/hydration.

DAY 104: **MASSIVE BONUS REST DAY!**

tick box

```
Week 15: Saturday: _ _ /_ _ /_ _
```

Woke up at: _ _ /_ _ am/pm
In bed now: _ _ /_ _ am/pm

Today I ate: OK ☐ WELL ☐ AWESOME ☐
My water intake was: OK ☐ GOOD ☐ AWESOME ☐
As a human I was: KIND ☐ THOUGHTFUL ☐ PRESENT ☐

Tomorrow I aim to be 1% better at:

: ....
: ....
: ....

As I prepare to close my eyes
I am grateful for:

: ....
: ....
: ....

pen/pencil down
lights out
3 deep breaths

Only **15** days to go ➡ ➡ ➡

DAY
LONG <u>105</u> RUN

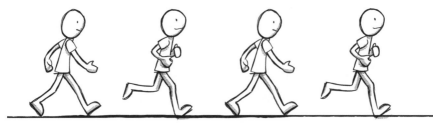

5 mins walk/60 mins easy run/ 5 mins walk/60 mins easy run
= 2 hrs 10 mins total

DOC YELLING SAYS: Remember, people run at different paces so distance covered may be different. Run continuously for 120 minutes if you're confident to do so.

YOUR FIFTEENTH LONG-RUN DAY!

LONG RUN NUMBER 15

Location: ....

Weather: ....

Time start: _ _ /_ _ am/pm

Time finish: _ _ /_ _ am/pm

Mood before: ....

Mood after: ....

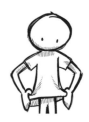

REMEMBER
TO WEAR
YOUR OFFICIAL
RACE-DAY TOP!

WRITE DOWN FIVE WORDS TO DESCRIBE YOUR DAY TODAY:

1. ....
2. ....
3. ....

4. ....
5. ....

DAY 105: HOMING IN!

tick box

Week 15: Sunday: _ _ /_ _ /_ _

NIGHTY NIGHT WEEK 15

Woke up at: _ _ /_ _ am/pm
In bed now: _ _ /_ _ am/pm

This week my diet has been OK ☐ PRETTY GOOD ☐ AWESOME ☐

This week I have slept OK ☐ WELL ☐ AMAZINGLY ☐

This week my training has gone OK ☐ WELL ☐ AWESOMELY ☐

Going into WEEK 16 I will:

1. Check in on my race pace and target time YES ☐ NO ☐

2. Feel free and at ease to alter it if it makes me feel at all uncomfortable YES ☐ NO ☐

3. Enjoy and celebrate my last Saturday training session YES ☐ NO ☐

As I prepare to close my eyes at the end of WEEK 15, I am grateful for:

1 ....

2 ....

3 ....

Next week in my training I aim to be 1 PER CENT better at:

....

pen/pencil down, lights out, 3 deep breaths

WEEK 15 OFFiCiALLY SMASHED ☐

tick box

Week 16

DiG DEEP WEEK!

AT A GLANCE:

Tues: 30 mins EASY RUN

Thurs: 50 mins EASY RUN/RACE PACE/
FASTER THAN RACE PACE/EASY RUN

Sat: 40 mins EASY RUN

Sun: 75 mins EASY RUN

TOTAL TRAINING TIME: 3 hrs 15 mins

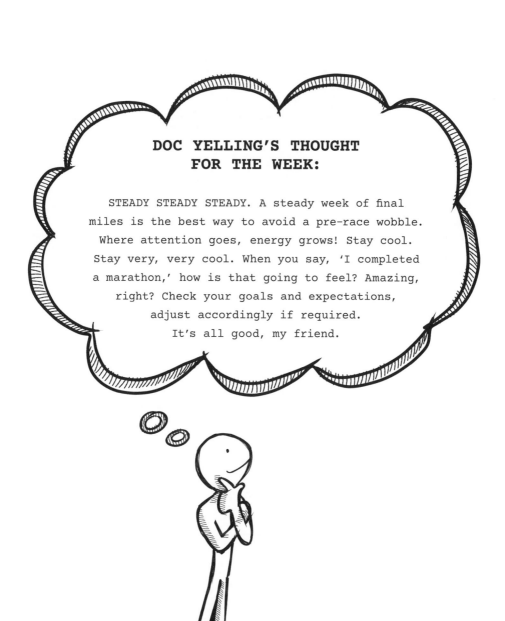

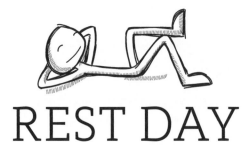

REST DAY

DON'T

THINK

ABOUT RUNNING

OR

ANYTHING

TO

DO

WITH

RUNNING

AT

ALL

(SEE YOU TOMORROW)

DAY 106: **MAGIC!**

tick box

Week 16: Monday: _ _ /_ _ /_ _

Woke up at: _ _ /_ _ am/pm
In bed now: _ _ /_ _ am/pm

Today I ate: OK ☐ WELL ☐ AWESOME ☐
My water intake was: OK ☐ GOOD ☐ AWESOME ☐
As a human I was: KIND ☐ THOUGHTFUL ☐ PRESENT ☐

Tomorrow I aim to be 1% better at:

: ....
: ....
: ....

As I prepare to close my eyes
I am grateful for:

: ....
: ....
: ....

pen/pencil down
lights out
3 deep breaths

Only **13** days to go ➧➧➧➧

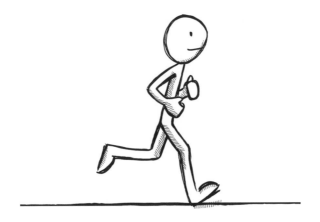

30 mins easy run

NOTES:

Location: ....

Weather: ....

Time start: _ _ /_ _ am/pm

Time finish: _ _ /_ _ am/pm

DAY 107: **GET iN THERE!**

tick box

```
┌─────────────────────────────────────────┐
│  Week 16: Tuesday: _ _ /_ _ /_ _         │
└─────────────────────────────────────────┘
```

Woke up at: _ _ /_ _ am/pm
In bed now: _ _ /_ _ am/pm

Today I ate: OK ☐ WELL ☐ AWESOME ☐

My water intake was: OK ☐ GOOD ☐ AWESOME ☐

As a human I was: KIND ☐ THOUGHTFUL ☐ PRESENT ☐

Tomorrow I aim to be 1% better at:

: ....
: ....
: ....

As I prepare to close my eyes
I am grateful for:

: ....
: ....
: ....

pen/pencil down
lights out
3 deep breaths

Only **12** days to go ➡➡➡➡

DAY
108

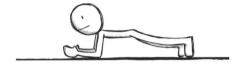

Rest Day/X-Train Day

If this was a theatre production heading into its final week of previews, the director would be doing anything and everything within their power to ensure the opening night goes with a bang. How about you do the same?

F.W.I.W.: Here's what I'm going to do:

1. Book a massage sometime in the next week.

2. Check how my tummy feels about my target finish time/race pace.

3. Re-do the maths of when/where I need to be around the course to achieve the above comfortably WHILE REMEMBERING TO ENJOY EVERY STEP.*

4. Figure out when/how to change strategy mid-race should I need to. (Much less complicated than it sounds and really good for confidence.)

5. Make sure I'm happy with my plan B. Make sure I actually have a plan B!!

* I always aim to run 10:30 mins/mile for the first 10 miles, 11:00 for the second 10 miles, which leaves me some wriggle room of 12:30, should I need it, for the last six miles. This 'usually' gets me in under 5 hours.

KEEP FOCUSED ... KEEP IT FUN ... KEEP ON KEEPIN' ON ...

DAY 108: TOTALLY PERFORMED!

tick box

Week 16: Wednesday: _ _ /_ _ /_ _

Woke up at: _ _ /_ _ am/pm
In bed now: _ _ /_ _ am/pm

Today I ate: OK ☐ WELL ☐ AWESOME ☐
My water intake was: OK ☐ GOOD ☐ AWESOME ☐
As a human I was: KIND ☐ THOUGHTFUL ☐ PRESENT ☐

Tomorrow I aim to be 1% better at:

: ....
: ....
: ....

As I prepare to close my eyes
I am grateful for:

: ....
: ....
: ....

pen/pencil down
lights out
3 deep breaths

Only 11 days to go ➡ ➡ ➡ ➡

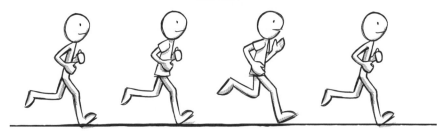

10 mins easy run/
20 mins race pace/
10 mins faster than race pace/
10 mins easy run
= 50 mins total

NOTES:

Location: ....

Weather: ....

Time start: _ _ /_ _ am/pm

Time finish: _ _ /_ _ am/pm

DAY 109: **WALLOPED!**

tick box

```
Week 16: Thursday: _ _ /_ _ /_ _
```

Woke up at: _ _ /_ _ am/pm
In bed now: _ _ /_ _ am/pm

Today I ate: **OK** ☐ WELL ☐ AWESOME ☐

My water intake was: **OK** ☐ GOOD ☐ AWESOME ☐

As a human I was: KIND ☐ THOUGHTFUL ☐ PRESENT ☐

Tomorrow I aim to be 1% better at:

: ....
: ....
: ....

As I prepare to close my eyes
I am grateful for:

: ....
: ....
: ....

pen/pencil down
lights out
3 deep breaths

Only **10** days to go ➡ ➡ ➡ ➡

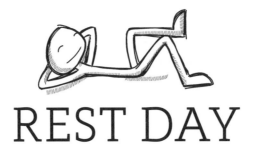

REST DAY

FUN FRIDAY, PRE-RACE WEEK,
CITY MARATHON SUPER HACKS:

THREE THINGS NO ONE TOLD ME ABOUT RUNNING THE LONDON MARATHON
FOR THE FIRST TIME - BEFORE I WAS ACTUALLY RUNNING IT!!

1. Watch out for speed bumps, kerbs and road furniture in the
first few miles; 47,000 people bunched up is brilliant for the
human spirit and an amazing phenomenon to experience, but it
means you can barely see the ground beneath your feet.

2. If you think you might want to take on some fluid at the next
drinks station, begin to think about positioning yourself where
you will need to be on the course well in advance. It's so easy
to leave it too late, get stuck in the pack and miss a much
needed splash and dash of revitalising and refreshing hydration.

3. Be prepared for your running watch to buzz each mile a little
earlier than the on-course mile markers come up. The 26 miles
385 yards official distance is digitally measured as a perfect
line from start to finish. Everyone always ends up running a wee
bit further but don't worry, the adrenaline more than makes up
for the required extra few yards.

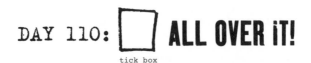

DAY 110: **ALL OVER iT!**

tick box

```
Week 16: Friday: _ _ /_ _ /_ _
```

Woke up at: _ _ /_ _ am/pm
In bed now: _ _ /_ _ am/pm

Today I ate: OK ☐ WELL ☐ AWESOME ☐
My water intake was: OK ☐ GOOD ☐ AWESOME ☐
As a human I was: KIND ☐ THOUGHTFUL ☐ PRESENT ☐

Tomorrow I aim to be 1% better at:

: ....
: ....
: ....

As I prepare to close my eyes
I am grateful for:

: ....
: ....
: ....

pen/pencil down
lights out
3 deep breaths

Only **9** days to go ➡ ➡ ➡ ➡

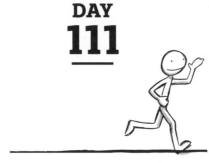

40 mins easy run

HEY FRIEND,

So here we are, we've arrived at our first 'last' of the next few days. This is our last Saturday run before the race, the ultimate rest-day RACE-DAY EVE.

Take time today, perhaps even a whole coffee's worth of reflection on what you have achieved over the last 16 weeks. Look back and meditate on how far you've come, all the different places and conditions you've run in, and how much you've learned about yourself.

You should be extremely proud. Like, really, really proud. Perhaps even give yourself permission to shed a quiet, little tear of JOY, FULFILMENT AND GRATITUDE. Have I told you lately that

YOU'RE AWESOME!!

Later this evening, while in bed, leaf back through this journal, YOUR JOURNAL, to revisit all your runs, when/where/how you felt, before/after. The Saturday runs have always been the signature runs for me ahead of the big Sunday push. They are where everything comes together.

We love Saturdays!!

Here's to you and here's to our last Saturday running day together. (FOR NOW!!)!)

DAY 111: BYE BYE, OLD FRIEND!

ONE MORE COCONUT FLAT WHITE, FOR OLD TIME'S SAKE!

tick box

Week 16: Saturday: _ _ /_ _ /_ _

Woke up at: _ _ /_ _ am/pm
In bed now: _ _ /_ _ am/pm

Today I ate: OK ☐ WELL ☐ AWESOME ☐
My water intake was: OK ☐ GOOD ☐ AWESOME ☐
As a human I was: KIND ☐ THOUGHTFUL ☐ PRESENT ☐

Tomorrow I aim to be 1% better at:

: ....
: ....
: ....

As I prepare to close my eyes
I am grateful for:

: ....
: ....
: ....

pen/pencil down
lights out
3 deep breaths

Only 8 days to go ➡➡➡➡

LONG DAY 112 RUN
DAY
112

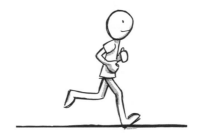

75 mins easy run
(including a few miles, no more
than five, at target race pace)

REHEARSE: Who are the people that are so special to you, the mere thought of whom will spur you on to the finish line? Dedicate each one of your five miles at race pace to them today and make a commitment to do the same for the last five miles of the race next Sunday.

LONG RUN NUMBER 16

Location: ....

Weather: ....

Time start: _ _ /_ _ am/pm

Time finish: _ _ /_ _ am/pm

Mood before: ....

Mood after: ....

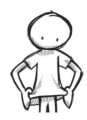

REMEMBER
TO WEAR
YOUR OFFICIAL
RACE-DAY TOP!

WRITE DOWN FIVE WORDS TO DESCRIBE YOUR DAY TODAY:

1. ....
2. ....
3. ....

4. ....
5. ....

DAY 112: iN SiGHT!

tick box

Week 16: Sunday: _ _ /_ _ /_ _

NIGHTY NIGHT WEEK 16

Woke up at: _ _ /_ _ am/pm
In bed now: _ _ /_ _ am/pm

This week my diet has been OK ☐ PRETTY GOOD ☐ AWESOME ☐

This week I have slept OK ☐ WELL ☐ AMAZINGLY ☐

This week my training has gone OK ☐ WELL ☐ AWESOMELY ☐

Going into MARATHON WEEK I will:

1. Know that I am awesome YES ☐

2. Give thanks to Doc Yelling YES ☐

3. REMEMBER TO ENJOY EVERY SECOND YES ☐

As I prepare to close my eyes at the
end of WEEK 16, I am grateful for:

1 ....

2 ....

3 ....

Next week in my training I aim to be
1 PER CENT better at:

....

pen/pencil down, lights out, 3 deep breaths

WEEK 16 OFFICIALLY SMASHED

tick box

Week 17

THiS iS iT!

AT A GLANCE:

Tues: 40 mins EASY RUN

Thurs: 30 mins EASY RUN

Sun: RACE DAY!!

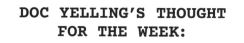

**DOC YELLING'S THOUGHT
FOR THE WEEK:**

Check the rearview mirror, look how far you've come.
What a supreme effort. Make the most of how all of this
feels, now and for the whole of the rest of your pre-race
week. How can something feel so amazing, petrifying,
nerve-racking and full of so much uncertainty all at
once? It's actually hilarious! All emotion is energy;
convert all of yours into race-day rocket juice.
STAY COOL. STAY VERY, VERY COOL.

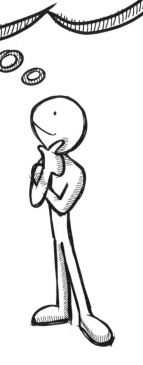

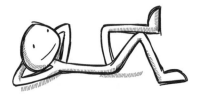

BE

NICE

TO

YOURSELF

DAY ONE

DAY 113: ☐ **TOO GOOD!**

tick box

Week 17: Monday: _ _ /_ _ /_ _

Woke up at: _ _ /_ _ am/pm
In bed now: _ _ /_ _ am/pm

Today I ate: OK ☐ WELL ☐ AWESOME ☐
My water intake was: OK ☐ GOOD ☐ AWESOME ☐
As a human I was: KIND ☐ THOUGHTFUL ☐ PRESENT ☐

Tomorrow I aim to be 1% better at:

: ....
: ....
: ....

As I prepare to close my eyes
I am grateful for:

: ....
: ....
: ....

pen/pencil down
lights out
3 deep breaths

Only 6 days to go ➡➡➡➡

BE

NICE

TO

YOURSELF

DAY TWO

Plus the small matter of a

40 mins easy run

(which your legs and your psyche will love
you for, but remember E-A-S-Y).

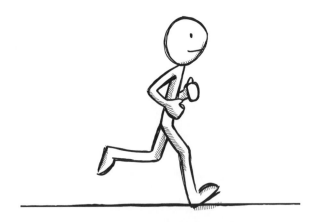

E-A-S-i-L-Y TiCKED AND EVERYTHING! BOOM!!

DAY 114:

tick box

Woke up at: _ _ /_ _ am/pm
In bed now: _ _ /_ _ am/pm

Today I ate: OK ☐ WELL ☐ AWESOME ☐
My water intake was: OK ☐ GOOD ☐ AWESOME ☐
As a human I was: KIND ☐ THOUGHTFUL ☐ PRESENT ☐

Tomorrow I aim to be 1% better at:

: ....
: ....
: ....

As I prepare to close my eyes
I am grateful for:

: ....
: ....
: ....

pen/pencil down
lights out
3 deep breaths

Only 5 days to go ➡ ➡ ➡

DAY
115

BE

NICE

TO

YOURSELF

DAY THREE

BONUS MARATHON MONK THINK:

The half-life of negative thoughts is extremely short, practically non-existent.

The only way a negative thought can survive beyond its first moment, is if we engage with it and turn it into an emotion.

If we pause, don't react and don't engage, whenever a negative thought arises, it will crumple and die before our very eyes.

Negative thoughts are chancers, they are fly-by-nights, they are snake-oil salesmen, travelling from door to door, looking for a patsy. DON'T BE THAT PATSY! DON'T ANSWER THE DOOR!!

If they knock again, wait it out. The knocking will cease.

Negative thoughts have no plan beyond the knock.

They have nothing in their locker,
other than the knocker.

Negative thoughts have not 'done the work'.

YOU HAVE DONE THE WORK.

DAY 115:

□
tick box

POSITIVELY
SMASHED!

```
Week 17: Wednesday: _ _ /_ _ /_ _
```

Woke up at: _ _ /_ _ am/pm
In bed now: _ _ /_ _ am/pm

Today I ate: **OK** ☐ WELL ☐ AWESOME ☐
My water intake was: **OK** ☐ GOOD ☐ AWESOME ☐
As a human I was: KIND ☐ THOUGHTFUL ☐ PRESENT ☐

Tomorrow I aim to be 1% better at:

: ....
: ....
: ....

As I prepare to close my eyes
I am grateful for:

: ....
: ....
: ....

pen/pencil down
lights out
3 deep breaths

Only **4** days to go ➡ ➡ ➡

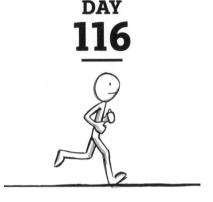

30 mins easy run

BE NICE TO YOURSELF DAY FOUR

PLUS: KEEP TAKING THE PRESSURE OFF RACE DAY

Prepare a checklist today for the weekend. Simple things like:

- Check weather.
- How many layers will you need while waiting at the start?
- Gloves? Hat? Sunnies?
- Podcast/playlist/both/neither?
- iPod/headphones charged?
- Gels/hydration?

The more admin/prep you can do ahead of race weekend, the more headspace you will have to relax and enjoy the wonder of all that hard work you've put in.

This sounds obvious but seriously, please take note. If you were having a dinner party, you wouldn't want to still be cooking, arranging the chairs and setting the table as the guests arrive. KEEP FRONT LOADING THOSE BASES IN YOUR RACE-DAY FAVOUR.

DAY 116: ¡ THANK YOU!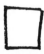

tick box

```
Week 17: Thursday: _ _ /_ _ /_ _
```

Woke up at: _ _ /_ _ am/pm
In bed now: _ _ /_ _ am/pm

Today I ate: OK ☐ WELL ☐ AWESOME ☐
My water intake was: OK ☐ GOOD ☐ AWESOME ☐
As a human I was: KIND ☐ THOUGHTFUL ☐ PRESENT ☐

Tomorrow I aim to be 1% better at:

: ....
: ....
: ....

As I prepare to close my eyes
I am grateful for:

: ....
: ....
: ....

pen/pencil down
lights out
3 deep breaths

Only **3** days to go ➡ ➡ ➡

DAY
117

THINGS PAULA RADCLIFFE TOLD ME THE FRIDAY BEFORE MY FIRST-EVER MARATHON

Don't over-eat in the next 48 hours. Carb loading is often blown up out of all proportion. (Paula told me this as we both tucked into a starter portion of mushroom risotto in the sunshine outside The Tower Hotel at Tower Bridge.)

Try to stay off your feet as much as possible between now and the start of the race. If you can, lie down. If you can't lie down, sit down. If you can't sit down, perch. If you can't perch, lean. If you can't lean, then stand but only for as little time as is absolutely necessary.

Once the race has started and you've settled down, after say a mile or so, ask yourself, 'Could I run faster if I wanted to?' If the answer is no, then you are already running too fast. In which case, slow down a bit, relax, recalibrate. THE NUMBER ONE MISTAKE OF FIRST-TIME MARATHON RUNNERS IS SETTING OFF TOO QUICKLY WITHOUT REALISING IT, BECAUSE YOU ARE TOO BLOODY EXCITED AND ARE HAVING THE MOTHER OF ALL ADRENALINE RUSHES.

Be ready for three mid-race dips, in fact, even better, expect them. Three periods where you have to tough it out. If they don't come – fantastic – but if they do, don't waste energy or focus by being surprised by them. Stay calm, STICK TO YOUR PLAN. They will pass. You will finish.

YOU HAVE DONE THE WORK

Try to get a good night's sleep. Box breathe. Sleep breathe. Slow down that heart rate. Think only good thoughts.

DAY 117: PAULA'S SUPER TiP DAY DONE BOOM!

tick box

Woke up at: _ _ /_ _ am/pm
In bed now: _ _ /_ _ am/pm

Today I ate: **OK** ☐ WELL ☐ AWESOME ☐
My water intake was: **OK** ☐ GOOD ☐ AWESOME ☐
As a human I was: KIND ☐ THOUGHTFUL ☐ PRESENT ☐

Tomorrow I aim to be 1% better at:

: ....
: ....
: ....

**As I prepare to close my eyes
I am grateful for:**

: ....
: ....
: ....

pen/pencil down
lights out
3 deep breaths

Only **2** days to go ➡➡➡➡

DAY
118

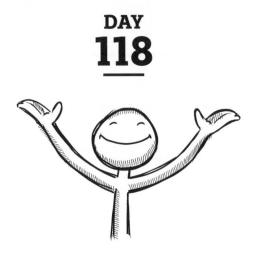

MARATHON EVE!

REMEMBER WHEN WE TALKED ABOUT THIS WAY BACK IN WEEK 1?

Well, now it's here, my friend. It's finally here. I love every Marathon Eve but nothing will ever beat the feeling of that first one. This is your first one. You lucky devil. I'm so JEALOUS.

This is your official welcome to the day before your marathon party. One of the most memorable days of your life. Because it's not just about tomorrow. It's about the rest of your life. What you're about to do in the next 24 hours will change you as a person forever. You will never be the same again. It's all going to be amazing. EVERY SINGLE MOMENT.

Because ...

YOU HAVE DONE THE WORK!!

P.S.: COMING UP, THE GREATEST MARATHON TIP OF ALL TIME. YES, I'VE LEFT THE BEST UNTIL LAST.

DAY 118: **WHAT A RiDE!**

tick box

Woke up at: _ _ /_ _ am/pm
In bed now: _ _ /_ _ am/pm

Today I ate: OK ☐ WELL ☐ AWESOME ☐
My water intake was: OK ☐ GOOD ☐ AWESOME ☐
As a human I was: KIND ☐ THOUGHTFUL ☐ PRESENT ☐

Tomorrow I aim to be 1% better at:

: ....

: ....

: ....

As I prepare to close my eyes
I am grateful for:

: ....

: ....

: ....

pen/pencil down
lights out
3 deep breaths

Only 1 day to go ➡ ➡ ➡

THE GREATEST MARATHON TIP OF ALL TIME

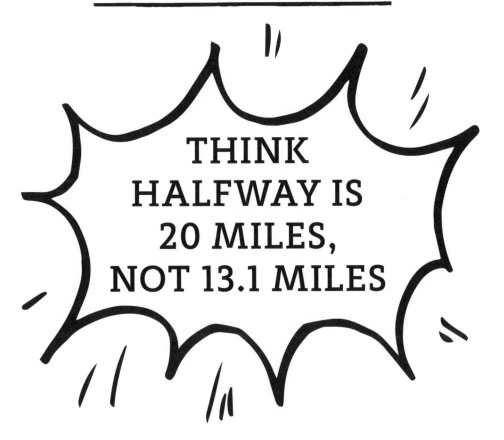

THINK HALFWAY IS 20 MILES, NOT 13.1 MILES

TRUST ME, IT'S LIKE MAGIC!! I know I have left this ridiculously late, but it doesn't work if you hear about it before now. Sorry!)

ONE MORE PAGE FOR LUCK

RUN WELL, MY FRIEND

STICK TO THE PLAN

GO FOR 'YOUR TIME'

DON'T SWEAT 'YOUR TIME'

SWEAT THE FUN

SWEAT THE EXPERIENCE

SWEAT 'THE WORK'

Right, I'm going to leave you in peace now. May I thank you for your company. I'm so profoundly pleased you chose to embark upon this amazing journey with me, this journal and my rambling amateur runner's thoughts. AFTER TOMORROW YOU WILL NEVER BE THE SAME AGAIN. Your amazing marathon experience will change your life forever. You are now a marathoner. All that's left to do is go collect your medal. It's approximately 26.2 miles away. Good luck. Run well. Stay safe. Be nice to yourself and all your fellow marathoners.

SEE YOU AT THE START LINE

Week 17: Sunday: _ _ /_ _ /_ _

RACE DAY
RACE DAY
RACE DAY

DOC YELLING SAYS:

Take a moment.
Stand confidently on the start line.
Look around, you've made it.
Reflect on how far you've come.
Close your eyes, breathe deeply, exhale slowly.

iT'S TiME TO RUN A MARATHON
BOOM BOOM BOOM!!

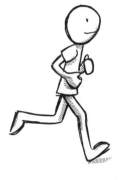

FOR LONDON MARATHON RUNNERS ONLY!

A PRICELESS LAST-MINUTE TAKEAWAY:

THE FIRST 6 MILES OF THE LONDON MARATHON HAS A LOT OF VERY FRIENDLY DOWNHILL SLOPES. THE COURSE FEEDS DOWN TOWARDS THE THAMES. THEY'RE NOT EXACTLY FOR FREE BUT THEY'RE PRETTY DARNED FRIENDLY! HALLELUJAH!

Location: ....

Weather: ....

Time start: _ _ /_ _ am/pm

Time finish: _ _ /_ _ am/pm

Mood before: ....

Mood after: ....

WRITE DOWN FIVE WORDS TO DESCRIBE YOUR DAY TODAY:

1. ....
2. ....
3. ....
4. ....
5. ....

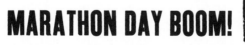

MARATHON DAY BOOM!

tick box

BOOM!

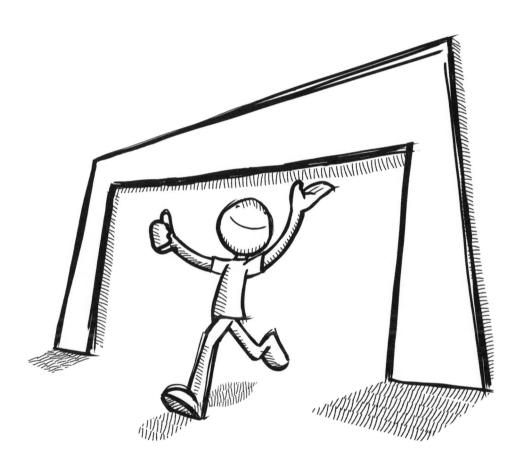

NOTES:

NOTES:

NOTES:

```
┌─────────────────────────────────┐
│           NOTES:                │
└─────────────────────────────────┘
```

NOTES:

NOTES:

NOTES:

NOTES:

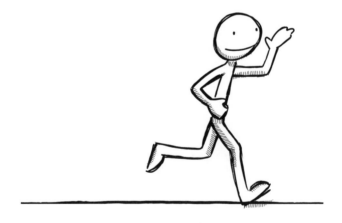